THE LIFE OF ALBERTO

Volume 2

Alberto E. Baston

The Life of Alberto
Volume Two

Story by Alberto E. Baston

Edited by Trenton Benard

Front Cover Painting by Tyler Koorndyk

Photography by Tyler Koorndyk and Erika Koorndyk

ISBN: Softcover   978-1-0820-9170-4

This book was printed in the United States of America.

To order additional copies of my books, website:

http://www.amazon.com/author/abaston

Dedication

I'm dedicating this book in loving memory of my father,
Norm Baston.

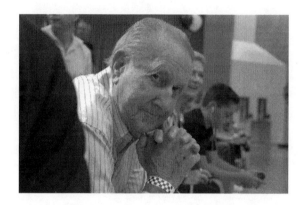

Norm Baston

_1930-2016_

Table of Contents

Chapter One:
Back In 1991

In the middle of July, my Grandma Vera came to California for a visit. This made me very glad. One day, I watched Grandma Vera write out postcards to her family at the kitchen table. One weekend while she was here, we went to Sophia's 100th birthday party. Sophia is Nana's mother, and a great grandma to Debbie and Gary. She was a very special woman. There was a huge party held outdoors, with music and a horseshoe game. Gary and my dad, Norm, played the horseshoe game. They had a good time. I was able to observe Sophia's huge family tree and learn from the pictures displayed inside of the house. This was a great party.

I turned 21 on my birthday. Danielle and I had a joint birthday party. She would turn 7 on August 14. We had a great birthday party with my family and Chico, one of Erika's first friends. He was a good guy.

The day after our party, Grandma Vera went back to Florida. She was done traveling for the time being. The long flight seemed to take a toll on her. I decided that I'd visit her in Florida. She was very happy when she heard this.

Near the end of July, my mom and I went to Irvine Valley College so that I could enroll. I signed up for four classes that would commence in the fall: Pre-Algebra (math), Adaptive Computer Assessment, Math Tutorial Lab and Writing. My classes were to start in October. I also signed up for OCTA Express and TRIPS, programs that were supposed to help me to be more mobile.

I was not excited to go to the college alone. It was a new level of education, a new experience in my life, and I knew it would be different than my other schools.

Before school started in the fall, my parents and I went to Florida for a few days in August. We stayed at my grandparents Gagan and Mamama's house. My grandparents were already in Alabama for Judd and Hena Te's wedding. Everybody was excited for their wedding. We flew to Birmingham, Alabama to join in the festivities. We stayed at my Uncle Puncho and Aunt Beba's house. Many relatives and friends came and visited. Hena Te and Judd were both very excited for the next day, the day that they would be married.

In the evening, we went to Trussville and held a rehearsal for their wedding. Then we went to a rehearsal dinner at a restaurant close to the church. We had a very good time.

August 10, 1991 was a beautiful wedding day for Hena Te and Judd. The wedding was a wonderful event. They were a loving couple, and they had a surprise for me after the wedding. We went to another room in the church. They wanted me to witness the signing of their wedding certificate.

I signed my name on it! They were highly excited for me. Later, we went to the wedding brunch at the clubhouse. It looked like a library or a courthouse. I enjoyed their wedding.

Then, we went back to Miami. I was excited for a road trip to the Disney amusement parks. Tia Maricosa drove her SUV to Orlando for four hours. On the first night, Tia Maricosa, Mimi, my parents and I went to Walt Disney World Magic Kingdom. I didn't know this park was larger than Disneyland. We visited Tomorrowland and rode the Carousel of Progress. It was an animated show with robots all about lifestyle, electronics and gadgets that we've utilized from the 1920s into the future. It was a so-so show. We rode the PeopleMover. It was a little different than the one at Disneyland. Then we went to Fantasyland.

We saw the Country Bears Jamboree. I loved it. We saw animatronic bears play country music! Then we walked around Fantasyland. We saw Mickey Mouse's Barn, and it looked like Toontown from Disneyland. I had a wonderful night. We went back to the resort to rest.

On the next day, Gagan and Mamama came down from Alabama to join us. We all went to Epcot. It was a theme park featuring science, life, nature, and various popular countries. I had a fan hat to keep cool with. We rode the Spaceship Earth ride. It detailed the history of invention all the way thru to the future. I loved it. Next was Journey into Imagination. It was certainly a crazy and imaginative ride. I liked Figment, the little dragon from the ride. We went to Canada, the United Kingdom, France, Morocco, Japan, the American Adventure, Italy, Germany, China, Norway and Mexico, all at Epcot. I enjoyed all the countries. We went on The Gran Fiesta Tour ride in (Epcot's) Mexico. It was about Mexico and the Three Caballeros. It looked like the ride *"It's a Small World"*. We went to see the stores in a few countries.

A few minutes later, a little rain began to come down. We were inside of the store in either Norway or Germany. The rain stopped. We went to The Land. It was a boat ride all about plants, fishes, and foods from plants. We loved it.

Then, we went to the worst show about food that I've ever seen. The Foods Rock was a rock and roll music show all about, you guessed it: food.

We went to The Living Seas. It was an aquarium. I liked it. Then we went to the best ride ever: The Universe of Energy. It was about energy and dinosaurs, and we were shown movies about energy. It was very different from all the other rides. My father loved it too. We went to the Wonders of Life. It was about life and biology. I thought this one was ok. The Universe of Energy was a hard act to follow.

Finally, we went to Horizon. This ride was about living life and utilizing gadgets in the future. I liked it. Epcot was the best park ever. We went back to the resort and slept.

On the next day, my grandparents went back to Miami. Our remaining family went to Disney-MGM Studios (which since then has become known as Disney Hollywood Studios). It was a huge theme park that reminded me of Universal Studios. We went to see the Indiana Jones Action Show. I liked the show. We went on the bus tour to check out some behind-the-scenes action from film and tv shows. This was fun. We went to The Animation. It was very interesting, and I enjoyed it. I wished to be an artist or animator.

We went to "*Honey, I Shrunk the Kids*". There were big plants, big mushrooms, and a giant fake ant. Afterward, we got lunch.

After lunch, we went to Muppet Vision 4D. It was awesome! In 4d, we felt the air blowing from behind, got a little wet from splashes and could see and touch real bubbles. I thought this was amazing.

Lastly, we went to The Great Movie Ride. It was an excellent ride featuring scenes from old westerns, Terminator, Alien and The Wizard of OZ (the live action version). I loved it.

On the next day, we flew back to Miami. We stayed there for a few more days before flying back to California. Home, sweet home.

Finally, October arrived. It was my first day of attendance to Irvine Valley College. I had planned to take my scooter, but it was under maintenance (and the battery had died anyway). Instead, my mom gave me a ride and dropped me off near my pre-algebra class. I was very shy, though I still took a front row seat.

The class had about forty students and it was larger than my high school class of twenty. I liked this class. The professor was very friendly. After class, my mom picked me up and took me home.

The next day, I got my scooter back. I used bus transportation and loaded my scooter onto the bus to the college at 8:30 am. My pre-algebra course was at 10:30 am, but today I had another class before that one. I went inside of the building, found the door and saw a note that said my writing class had been canceled. I was rather shocked that this happened.

While waiting for my next class, I cruised around the college on my scooter. I went to the bookstore to browse. Soon it was time, so I went outside and went to my pre-algebra class.

After class, I waited for my bus at 12:30 pm. The bus took me home. Sometimes though, my bus wouldn't show up. I'd wait for 15 minutes beyond the schedule and then I'd call my mom via pay phone to pick me up. I hated when this happened, and it happened to me quite a few times. I became furious with public transit and wanted to throw the bus into the ocean (with no people inside!).

On October 26, I met my first grand-nephew Joey Guccione. Alicia became a big sister for the first time. Michelle gained a new child. Sister Debbie gained a new grandchild!

On the weekend, I went to see Joey at their house. He was a good baby boy. I was very excited to meet him.

On the first Saturday of November, my parents went out of town with Jack and Marge. The Belchers were very good friends to my parents. They all went to Arizona. I stayed home with Totica. I had been invited to Carl Harvey School's Christmas party at the Marriott in Irvine. Then something happened to me. I will tell you about it in a bit. At 10.30 am, a bus from OCTA picked me up to go to Irvine Marriott.

I saw my old school friends. They were excited to see me. They performed Christmas songs. The party went very well until 1 pm. I saw a sign that said Bob Hope's birthday party tonight. That was cool.

Outside, I waited for my ride. The OCTA bus did not show up. I was very disappointed with the bus company again. I walked back inside. I stayed with Mr. Perez and Linda Perez, and they took me home around 3pm. I thought this was very nice of them. Totica had been very worried about me though.

In November, I went to a movie at the mall in Palm Desert. I saw Disney's Beauty and the Beast. The theater was almost full. I was sitting to the right in the front row. The movie was great, one of the best animated musicals ever.

On December 26, we went to Big Bear for post-Christmas family festivities. We rented a big house for 5 days. There was lots of snow and the air was freezing cold. The house had 2 rooms downstairs and a master bedroom upstairs. I hated the cold weather however I liked the snow. Everybody came together for our Christmas celebrations. I was excited to be in a house with a big satellite dish TV. I watched channels from the east coast and all over the world.

Debbie's family stayed at the house with us. Gary's family had another house 15 minutes away. My dad took a video of me standing at the window from outside. He said, *"Mr. Bates is at the window."* Norman Bates is a character from the movie *Psycho*. I didn't find this as funny as my dad did. Brittany, Lindsay and Danielle were riding the sleds down the small slopes of snow. They had lots of fun. Erika threw a few snowballs to my mom during the video. Danielle tried to throw a snowball at my mom too, but she fell.

Erika built a snowman outside. It almost looked like Olaf from the 2013 movie *Frozen*. I stayed inside and watched them. They had a blast. We had a great dinner that night. Michelle's family joined us the next morning. Joey was a good baby. I had to watch him for a bit. He was 3 months old. Alicia was 1 year old. She was a good girl.

Later that day, Gary's family joined us as well. The girls had fun sliding down the stairs. I know that it is dangerous to slide on stairs, but they all avoided any injury. We had a great time. On the next day, we went to the village for a walk and a round of shopping at the stores. The weather was both sunny and chilly, so 40 degrees felt like 20 degrees. We had fun.

On the next day, Debbie's family and Michelle's family left for home. Gary's family stayed with us until the night. In the middle of the night, my parents and I heard a snowstorm. My mom was excited to see so much snow fall. We went back to sleep.

On the next day, we were packing and cleaning the house. I went outside and saw a cute squirrel. The squirrel was hiding its nut, retrieving it and then picking another spot to hide the same nut. It did this a few times.

It was the last day to play in the snow. My mom and I rode the sled. It was good fun, but I couldn't get up in the snow. We got up and walked up the hill, then fell in the snow. We laughed together. Honestly, I was terrified. I got up and knocked Erika's snowman's nose off. We went back to home. It was the best Christmas vacation ever.

Chapter Two:
1992

In the spring of 1992, I went to my old schools for quick visits to my teacher Mrs. Dunn and my friend Melissa. They were doing fine, and they were excited to see me. I was excited to see them too. They had relocated to Valley High School. Carl Harvey School was going to change to an Elementary School and add kids without disabilities in the fall of 1992. This was disappointing. I liked our old campus.

I had a wild rabbit in my backyard. I named this rabbit Boo. Boo came around for about six weeks before I fed them. I held a carrot between my fingers, and Boo seemed to think about taking it. They came closer to me, and then, Boo took the carrot out of my hand! Then they jumped back a couple of feet. It became a wonderful memory. I didn't yet know that Boo was a female rabbit. I would find out a few weeks later. Boo showed up again, and this time she had a baby bunny with her. They were cute. They shared carrots and played together. I was so happy that I laughed like Goofy. This was the last time I'd see them. I would miss them long after they were gone.

On the weekends in Palm Desert, I'd go to the swimming pool when the weather was hot. I loved to swim, and I loved the little diving area by the step. I did this almost every weekend. It was very fun.

One day, I wanted to see the movie "Batman Returns", the second Batman movie, at the Palm Desert Theater. My mom told me, *"You don't need to pay,"* and she dropped me off. The guy at the front asked, *"Where's your ticket?"* I pointed my left thumb back. *"Ok,"* he said. I went inside. I felt embarrassed, but no matter. I was going to see my movie.

The ticket guy followed me, and he told me, *"After the movie, you will pay for a ticket."* After the movie was over, I saw another guy at the door. I exited and walked away and waited for my mom to pick me up. She was right, I didn't need to pay anything.

At night, on the weekends, my parents would go out to eat for dinner. I would get a little bored, so I would watch TV and play games on my Nintendo.

Some nights, I would turn music on and perform songs by New Kids on the Block, Jon Secada and Michael Bolton, all by myself. I often lip-sang and danced while my parents went out at dinner. I never told anyone.

On Easter Weekend, everybody came to Palm Desert to celebrate with us. We packed 15 people into one condo house. Anywhere you looked, someone had made a bed of any open space there was- air mattresses, the couch, and the sofa were all employed. I slept on an air mattress in my parents' room. Everybody enjoyed our arrangements.

We went to the pool. I had fun with Danielle, Brittany and Lindsay. My father, Tom and Gary went to play golf. In the evening, as I was eating my dinner, a bird entered the house. The bird flew into the kitchen and then into the living room. Somebody caught the bird and went outside to let it fly free.

Later, Gary, Tom and my dad were playing a game of poker on the patio. My mom wanted to scare my dad, so she hid a frog in the money bag. While my dad went to the bathroom, my mom caught the unaware frog from the golf course and hid it in the money bag.

My dad came back, and someone asked him to check the bag. He grabbed the bag and opened it.

When the frog jumped out at him, my dad got scared and jumped. He said a bad s-word a few times. Everybody burst into laughter. It was very much the funniest moment ever. I love my father.

On Easter Day, the guys went to play some golf. The rest of us went to the church. The church was full up. Unlike our condo, the church was not fun when it was so crowded. We went back to the house. My mom and I got Easter eggs to hide at the pool area. While we were hiding them, I dropped an Easter egg in the grass. Then we went back to the house and gathered the kids for an Easter Egg Hunt. They had a blast.

We walked to the clubhouse for Easter Brunch. We took our family pictures at the front of the clubhouse. I had already had my lunch before we went to the clubhouse, so I just hung out. Then, after lunch, everybody prepared to go back home. Easter Day went well.

That summer, on a Thursday, I went to Lake Havasu, Arizona. My mom drove us there, and it took four hours! We dropped our things off at the hotel we were staying at.

Then, we met Gary's family at his trailer near the river. On Friday, I got on the boat. Gary drove the boat atop the Colorado River. Somewhere in the river, Lindsay and Brittney were swimming in the cold water, and doing very well at it. They had a lot of fun. I tried going in the water, but it was the most freezing thing I had ever touched. It felt like a lake in Alaska!! I decided to never get back in that water.

After that, I went to the London Bridge, Arizona to check out different shops with Cyndee, Brittney and Lindsay.

In the evening, I went back to Gary's trailer for dinner. Brittney, Lindsay and I watched The Three Stooges, The Little Rascals, and Elvis videos on their TV. We had a lot of fun.

Late in the afternoon that Saturday, I went to the casino in the best town to gamble in. It is not Las Vegas. It is Laughlin,

Nevada. I went to the Flamingo hotel to stay one night and play the casino games for the first time ever. I was highly excited. Gary was the one who had told me the Flamingo casino was better than Las Vegas. That night, I went and played the 25-cent slot machine for a half hour. I won $400 on that slot machine. I was very lucky. My parents were thrilled. But the cashier only paid me half of what I'd won. My mom said this was wrong.

Two security guards came, and they began to discuss the money with my mom. They thought that my mom was incorrect. Eventually, secretaries came and solved the problem. We were given $400 cash. Then, my mom and I went to the blackjack table for a few minutes. We played and won $100. We left the casino with more money than we came with and went to another hotel. My dad played the slot machine there, but he had no luck. We went back to the Flamingo hotel to sleep.

Can you guess what happened at 4:00 am in the morning? The window had begun to shake. I was not afraid. It was a small earthquake. I heard other people in the hallway, scared awake from the earthquake. I was still in bed, so I went back to sleep.

At 8:00 am, we had another surprise visitor. It was another small earthquake. The windows and beds shook for 30 seconds.

At 10:00 am, we checked out of the hotel and headed home. This was a thrilling weekend. I had $500 cash on hand and made deposits into my bank. I called this trip a success.

Sometimes in the summer, Brittney and Danielle would stay with us for a few days. We rode my scooter in front of my house. They had a great time.

In the evening, we went to Sizzler for dinner. I'll never forget what happened to me at Sizzler. I was wearing white pants. Danielle was sitting by me, and she spilled Coca Cola... right onto my pants. I felt embarrassed, but I was going to be ok.

In the fall, I attended two colleges. I took a computer drawing and an animation class at OCC in Costa Mesa on Tuesdays and Thursdays at 9:30 am and 11 am. I didn't like this college at all. The computer used *Amiga* to make animation. This was a bit difficult. I also hated that sometimes, I tried to open the door to class but could not, and so I knocked to get someone's attention. The door was too hard to open. Nobody could hear me (or at least, nobody answered). Because of this, I missed the animation class a few times. I was unhappy on this campus. When I did not make it into animation class, I'd go to the bookstore to read until my bus got back at 12:30 pm.

On Mondays and Wednesdays, I went to Irvine Valley College and took Algebra, Computer lab, Multimedia and Desktop Publishing. I liked computer lab, and I enjoyed making a slideshow of Disneyland's future sister park. It was called Westepcot (before being changed to Disney's California Adventure a few years later).

I liked this college better than the other one. However, I hated that there were times that the bus didn't show up to take me home! I'd go to the pay phone and call my mom to pick me up. I used my phone card to make the call. My mom would pick me up and take me home.

In October, my mom and I went to Michelle's house to babysit Alicia and Joey for a few hours. I loved them. We played with their toys. As I was picking up the toys to put them into their basket, cute little Joey helped me! I was very proud of him. This became a great memory.

One Saturday, we went to Disneyland for Erika's Goofy parade. Erika was in costume as Chip the chipmunk. She did a good job. Debbie's family came to see Erika's parade too. We were all proud of our chipmunk. Afterwards, we went on a few rides like It's a Small World and watched the Fantasmic show. Then, we went back home.

On Thanksgiving weekend, I went to the Desert house. Everyone joined us there. We went to the movie theater and saw Disney's Aladdin. I loved the genie and his voice by Robin Williams. We loved it. We went to go shopping at the mall and we saw an ice rink. I remembered my nieces loved to ice skate. They were good at skating. I loved to watch them.

16

In December, I went to my sister Debbie's house to celebrate Christmas eve. It was a good time. A special Santa came to entertain the kids. Then, we opened our presents. I got my first MasterCard credit card from my parents. I thought this was nice. It went good, Christmas that year.

Chapter Three:
1993

I went back to Irvine Valley College in the spring. I took a computer business course on Tuesday and Thursday afternoons. I liked this class, despite one thing: My bus came 15 minutes before my class was out. I let my professor know, and she told me that it was okay if I left early to catch the bus. I was relieved.

Still, sometimes the bus would not show up. Once again, I wanted to throw the bus into the ocean. I would get so mad that I felt like The Incredible Hulk.

Frank took me to the computer fair at UCI. He was very nice. We were looking at new stuff for computers. We did not buy anything, but we did have a great time.

On July 10, I went to Alabama for Cousin Mel-Marie's wedding. I met Chris. He's a good man, and at the time he was Mel-Marie's husband-to-be. The wedding was great, and the reception was too. The next day, I went back to California.

For the summer, I re-enrolled in Physical Education. I tried to do mat exercises, and my body made some crazy cracking sounds. After the mat exercises, I liked to use the hand bike for five minutes. After that, I liked to pull down the weight bar for twenty reps. I'd wrap it all up by walking on the treadmill for 10 minutes. I loved the treadmill the most. I had a great time at P.E.

My nieces Brittney and Danielle came and stayed with us for a week. One evening, we went back to Sizzler for dinner. Can you guess what happened to me at Sizzler? Danielle went and spilled coca cola onto my pants again. We couldn't keep ourselves from laughing. This was my favorite moment.

Another week, Lindsay stayed with us. She was a good, sweet niece. Linda, Elizabeth, Jessica, and Justin came back to California for a week. We went to the movies and saw the worst picture ever: *The Last Action Hero*. It was the dumbest action movie ever. The movie was about a boy who wanted to be in an action movie.

We picked up Danielle at her house and went to the Universal Studios Tour. This was the last time we'd take the Universal Studio Tour. It was a grand and expansive place. We went on the Back to the Future ride. It was a time travel ride in which we were transported to the time of the dinosaurs, evident by the scenery on the giant screen. It was a cool ride.

Then we went on the trams for a behind-the-scenes experience detailing the making of movies, tv shows and special effects, from floods of water to King Kong to the broken bridge to

Jaws to a dizzying tunnel. It was very cool. Then we had lunch, and then we went on the E.T. ride. It was awesome. We had a wonderful time at the Universal Studios. We dropped Danielle back off before heading home.

On the weekend we went to palm desert and enjoyed the swimming pool. We also went shopping at the mall where the girls liked to skate on ice. They had a great time. I had a great time in the pool.

On Sunday night, we went back home to Irvine. After a few days, Linda, Elizabeth, Justin and Jessica went back to Michigan. I loved them.

A few days later, I realized that I had lost my school ring. It had a ruby, a falcon emblem and my name. I didn't remember where my ring was. I was disappointed in myself.

In the fall, I met new desert friends. Bill and Donna are very good musicians. Bill was a great pianist. Donna was a sweet woman who loved teaching people about music and playing the piano. She also loved *The Phantom of The Opera.* They owned Desert Piano and Organ store in Palm Desert. They offered for my parents to join in on their local tv commercial. They made a funny commercial, and I think they did well. They had a great time. Bill and Donna had private performances, and they invited us to attend.

Later that weekend, Bill found my school ring at the pool. He returned my ring to me. I told him thank you. I was so excited to have my ring back.

I went back to my college. I took a music class, Basics of Music 1. I liked this class. Sometimes, after the class, I'd notice that the bus had not shaken its old habit- it wouldn't show up. I think you may have a decent idea of what I wanted to do to the bus. It's probably better for their sake that I didn't see them on these days.

A few days later, I saw a fire from Laguna Hills moving toward my hometown of Turtle Rock. My mom was so afraid that she couldn't sleep. At midnight, we stood out front with our neighbors Diane and Steve, watching the fire move up the hill. At 12:30, I went to bed in exhaustion and slept until 4am. The firemen had taken care of things.

Thanksgiving week, my parents and I went to Miami for the celebration of Tia Maricosa's 50th birthday party. The party was to take place at her house on Saturday night. We were staying at my grandparents Gagan and Mamama's house. On Thanksgiving Day, my parents and I went to aunt Connie's house in Fort Lauderdale to celebrate Thanksgiving with my dad's family; cousin Mark, Judy, Liz, Paul and grandma Vera. We had a wonderful time. Then we went back to Miami.

On Saturday evening, we went to Tia Maricosa's 50th birthday party. A lot of family joined us, including cousins Mark and Judy. We had a wonderful party.

My mom and I went to the bookstore en espanol in Miami for Totica's Christmas presents. I bought a book for her. A few days later, we went back to California.

In December, we took Cyndee and my nieces Brittney, Lindsay and Danielle to see the Nutcracker ballet at the Irvine Barclay theatre. They loved it.

My mom bought a used computer for Danielle for Christmas. I installed a few programs and games. I felt a small earthquake for something like five seconds as I was finishing her computer.

On Christmas Day, we celebrated Christmas with my family at my house. We had a Christmas dinner and an opening of the presents. Danielle was excited about the computer she received from us.

Chapter Four:
1994

I went back to my college at Irvine Valley College. I took Beginner's Piano 1, P.E., Acting 1 and Theatre Production 1. I liked the piano class. I found that it is easy to play the piano. I loved P.E. I did exercises on the hand cycling machine, pulled down the weight bar, and walked on the treadmill. I also lifted the 2.5lb weight.

I went to my acting class. I didn't speak in class. I learned acting in the style of Charlie Chaplin and Pilot and Janitor. A few weeks later, the teacher asked me to withdraw from this class. I dropped the class. Theatre production class was closed for the season, and I do not know why. I wished to be an actor in a sitcom or movie in the future. But, it's not easy acting.

My bus had gone from habitually abandoning me to an attitude of outright neglect. If I had seen that bus on these days, it might have gotten thrown all the way to another continent.

I took Danielle to see the famous magician David Copperfield at Segerstrom Center for the Arts. He did a few classic magic tricks, and some special tricks with his duck, Webster. He also showed us that he can fly. I couldn't see any wire attached to him, so as far as I'm concerned that guy can fly.

It was a good show, a particularly thrilling experience. We enjoyed our time at this show.

Then we went to eat dinner at a private club. They had good foods. I was surprised to see Danielle eat enough for two dinners. She was a good eater. We had the greatest night ever.

I went back to Palm Desert for Easter. Everybody came and joined us for a massive sleepover. I took Nana on the golf cart and drove around the streets and around the clubhouse. We had a great time. On Easter Day, we went to a different Catholic Church. The priest was very mean. It was bad. We went back to my desert house. My mom and I went to the pool area to hide the Easter eggs. We gathered the kids to hunt them down, and they had a great time. My dad, Gary and Tom came back from playing golf and we all walked to the clubhouse for Easter brunch. We had a good time. After brunch, we left Palm Desert to go home to Irvine. I hated the traffic.

I enrolled in P.E. again that summer and did the same exercises. I loved it.

We invited Brittney and Danielle to stay over with us for a week. One day, my mom and I took them to a horseback riding lesson at Coto de Caza. Danielle was extremely excited, and

Brittney felt ok about it. They both had a great time once we were there though.

Later in the summer, I had my niece Lindsay over for a week. We went to the movie theater and saw Disney's *The Lion King*. It was a very scary movie for Lindsay, but we enjoyed it. A few days later, I had my cousins Jeanina, Diana, Lisette and Patricia join up with Lindsay, my mom, and I. We went to Fashion Island to walk to the movie theater. We saw the worst movie ever. It was called *Baby's Day Out*. Lindsay had a great time, laughing louder than anyone else in the theater. Everybody loved her laughs. Lindsay loved this movie very much.

I went to visit my godmother's house. My cousin Diana taught me how to do a fortune teller reading with string and a needle. I asked her my spiritual question: How many babies will I have in the future? The needle answered first by moving forward and back, which means boy.

Second, the needle answered with a circle, which means girl. Last, the needle answered by moving forward and back, which meant boy again. I wished that I would have 3 kids in some future, somewhere. I didn't believe that my future hope would come true. I asked another question. Will I be famous? The needle answered forward and back, which mean yes. Will I have a girlfriend in this year? It answered with a circle, which means no. This much was true.

A few days later, my great uncle Tata died. It was a sad day. He made many jokes, and he made me happy. He was one of the greatest uncles ever. I felt sorry for my great aunt Bobbie. I asked my mom what I should wear for the funeral. I thought I needed darker glasses. My mom laughed, "It's not a movie." For some reason, I couldn't cry for my Uncle. I'm going to miss Tata.

A few weeks later, I went to the movie theater with Danielle, Brittney, my mom and her friend Amnery. We saw *Black Beauty*, a horse movie. I know you may think I am one of the toughest guys around, but at the end of the movie the whole theater could hear me crying. Everybody looked at me, bewildered. I stopped crying after two minutes. It was the saddest movie ever. But I still missed Tata.

In the fall, I went back to my college. I took an advanced (adaptive) grammar and writing class, and P.E. too. The grammar and writing class was not easy. I liked P.E. better.

I went back to Miami for Christmas and the New Year. I stayed at my grandparents' house. A few days later, my cousins Junior, Mimi, her boyfriend Carlos and I went to the movie theater (spoiler alert).

We saw *Star Trek Generations.* I hated that Captain Kirk died. Mimi cried. It was a sad movie, but we loved it. I liked Data.

I went to Tia Maricosa's house on Christmas Eve. We had a great dinner. Afterward, I saw my aunt cleaning the dishes as my grandma sang and danced in the kitchen. My mom was singing too. This was a beautiful moment.

We went to the living room to open the Christmas presents. I got a cigarette box with my name *'Prince Albert'* on it. We laughed. It was a weird present (I don't smoke cigarettes). My family continued to open their presents. We all had a great time.

On Christmas Day, my mom, dad and I went to Fort Lauderdale and visited Aunt Connie's house to celebrate Christmas with my dad's family. Grandma Vera was happy to see us.

Chapter Five:
1995

In January, my mom turned 50 years old. My dad threw her a grand party at the Century Club in Costa Mesa. Everybody came to my Mom's party. There was a harp player named Alfredo Ortiz playing during the evening's dinner portion. I thought he played well. After dinner, I sang a duet with Elton John of "Can You Feel the Love Tonight" from the movie *The Lion King*. Elton's parts were played back over cd. He must have been on the road because he hadn't responded to my e-mails. I must have sung well, because everyone started crying. My mom came to hug me. She was very proud of me. Then, everybody started dancing to Latin music by The Alturas. I danced a bit. We had a great time. The party was over at eleven.

The next day, my mom opened her birthday presents excitedly.

Marge and Jack Belcher took me to Cirque Du Soleil at the OC Fairground. I thought that it was nice of them to invite me. We enjoyed the show. I gave my truest thanks to Marge and Jack Belcher. I never forgot this moment in my life.

In the spring, I went back to my college. I took a Dynamics of Job Searching class. I had a mentor to help me with copying notes from the whiteboard. I did okay. I also took PE again. I spent a lot of time on the treadmill and got my speed up.

I enjoyed using the treadmill. On another day of the week, I took an MA intro to Windows class. It was too easy.

I went to two basketball games for Brittney and Lindsay. They were great basketball players, and I had a great time watching them. My brother Gary coached Brittney's team.

Cousin Ivette and I had movie dates at the theater a few times. I paid for her tickets. We had fun.

In the summer, I went back to Irvine Valley College and took PE again. I enjoyed it. Sometimes, before the class, I loved to watch the squirrel and the rabbit at the orange trees. I felt happy and peaceful.

In July we flew to Fort Lauderdale for my grandma Vera Baston's 95th birthday party ever. Once we arrived at the airport, we took a shuttle to the hotel. The hotel room wasn't to be ready until the morning, so we got a room somewhere else with Totica.

We went to Waffle House for dinner. Alicia said, "This place is disgusting!" We went back to the room. Totica and I both went to bed. I hated one thing: I could hear (clearly) through the wall that somebody was making big band hanky panky love sounds in the next room, and they didn't sound like they had plans to stop. I didn't sleep until 1:30 am.

In the morning, we got a suite with my parents. Grandma Vera joined us at the hotel, and we got her a suite too. She said, "I need a man." Everybody laughed. Our family went out for dinner.

My dad and I went back to Waffle House and got a waffle. I did not like it. It was hard and crispy. I ate it though. We went back to the suite and got ready before heading to the hotel's party room. We all celebrated Grandma Vera's 95th birthday together.

We danced to a few songs like Chicken Fingers, Macarena, and Celebration. We had a great party. Grandma Vera had the greatest birthday ever. A few days later, we went back to California.

In August, Tia Maricosa, Cousin Mimi and Cousin Junior came to California. My mom and her sister rode the balloon ride. Cousin Junior, Cousin Mimi and I went to Disneyland. We had a great time without our parents. We took a few rides, like Pirates of the Caribbean, Haunted Mansion, It's a Small World, Star Tours, and the monorail to the hotel before going home. Our parents were not back when we arrived. They showed up one hour later and let us know that they had had a great time.

I picked up Lindsay, Alicia, and Joey to spend time with us. In the car, Lindsay and Alicia were talking. Joey said, "Don't entertain me." I laughed at this so much. On the weekend, we went to Balboa Island. Lindsay went on the bungee jumper. She loved it. Alicia was a little too afraid to try it. She didn't do it. Later, when we were on the road headed home, Alicia said "I want to go on the bungee jumper next time."

I went back to school in the fall. I took an internet class in the computer lab. I also took P.E. again. I was enjoying school.

In December we went back to Big Bear to celebrate Christmas. My dad and Tom got a Christmas tree. We decorated the tree with help from my nieces Brittney, Danielle, and Lindsay. On Christmas Eve, we all enjoyed Christmas dinner together.

On Christmas morning we woke up to snow falling outside. Danielle went to the Christmas tree and opened her presents. We had a great time. Erika and Michelle's family came. Then Gary's family came too. Marge and Jack came for a visit with us. We had one of the greatest Christmases ever.

The next day, my mom took Brittney and Danielle to a skiing lesson. The weather was freezing, 30 degrees outside. I sat on the chair outside for an hour before they finished their lesson. What happened to me next? Two guys wanted me to try and ride on the special ski chair. I got on, and they got on the ski rail to go up and drop off the rail and ski down the mountain together with me. I felt like I was in a James Bond movie. I did this a few times for half an hour. I had the greatest skiing experience ever. If you two ever read this, thank you for taking me to have fun.

We went to Gary's cabin. I saw Brittney, Danielle and Lindsay, all three of them singing popular songs from TLC, and "Rudolph, the Red-Nosed Reindeer". They sang very well, although a little off pitch. I loved listening to them.

The next day, we went back home. We had one of the greatest Christmas vacations ever.

Chapter Six:
1996

I got my first chance to watch satellite tv from DirecTV, which was a little better than basic cable. Some channels were broadcast for the east coast. I loved to watch programs three hours earlier than the regular channels. It was the best service. I did not know how many channels were actually available on HBO, but there were a lot. Like, *a lot.*

My mom and I went to pick up her friends Astrid and Teresita from the hotel they were staying in. We went to my house and to Laguna Beach. We had a great time.

My mom wanted her best friend Amnery's 50th birthday party to be held at my house. Everybody came to my house. We had the greatest birthday party ever for Amnery.

I went back to my college. I took P.E. again. I was doing the same exercises as before. On a few occasions, the bus didn't show up to take me home. I felt weary about bus transportation. I wished to go back to the college with somebody as company in the future. I would not like to be alone at the college again. It's okay, though.

I went back to Palm Desert for Easter. Everybody came and joined us. We had a full house. We went to the pool and had a great time. We painted Easter eggs on the patio and played continental card games like gin rummy. I did not like to lose.

On Easter Day, my mom and I went to the church. Then, we went back to the house. Everybody was getting ready for Easter Brunch. My mom hid the Easter eggs at the patio and at the side house. The kids had a good time finding them. We went to the clubhouse for Easter Brunch. We took a few pictures together. We had a great time. Later that night, we went back home. I hated the traffic on the way home. It took us three hours to get back. Still, we had one of the greatest Easters ever.

We went to Las Vegas to meet my sister Linda. I went to The Luxor Hotel. I got on the elevator, and the elevator went sliding up in an interesting way that I wasn't used to. It was strange. On the first night, I went to The Sand Hotel for dinner. Then we went to a boring show about hypnotism. After the show, we talked with the lady about the show while we waited for my dad to get the car. She said, "I was actually just acting." I was surprised. We got back to The Luxor Hotel. On the next day, we picked Linda up from another hotel. We played the slot machines. I had no luck. Linda played bingo with her friends. We all had a great time. The next day, we visited my dad's friend Royce Shuya in Las Vegas. We had a good time with Royce.

My cousins Ivette and Johnny picked me up from the hotel. We went to Planet Hollywood. We went to try the slot machine, just one pull; and we had no luck. We went to Fido's workshop. I was glad to see Fido. Then, we went to Fido's house for a brief visit. Tati was excited to see me. Lisette was there too. They took me back to the hotel. I had a great time with them. Eventually, I went back home to California.

My parents, Jack, Marge and I went back to Miami. We were staying at my grandparents' house. I would sleep in my grandpa's recliner chair. My parents, Jack, and Marge left to Key West. I stayed between my grandparents' and my aunt's house. My grandpa took me to the bookstore.

While the red light was still on, he made a left turn on the red light when there was no traffic on the other side. I was shocked at my grandpa.

When we arrived at the bookstore. I bought a book for Totica. Then, we went back to my grandparents' house.

A few days later, my parents, Jack and Marge got back. We went to the restaurant to celebrate my grandparents' 55th anniversary. We had a great time. Another day, we went to visit my dad's sister Connie's house in Fort Lauderdale. I loved my grandma Vera's laughing. We went to a restaurant for lunch,

Mark and Judy joining us. We had a good time. Later, we went back to Miami. Another day, we went back home to California.

Sister Debbie took us to see Yanni's Concert at the Honda Center (the Anaheim Ducks' hockey stadium.) We had a good time. I loved his music with the electric pianos.

I went to see *Independence Day* at the movie theater. In it, aliens destroyed the earth, but Will Smith put a stop to the destruction and saved the world. This was a science fiction movie. I loved it. I watched it twice.

On July 4, I went to Teresita's house in Laguna Beach. We went to celebrate the 4th of July and also to celebrate Teresita's birthday. I did not like the steep uphill road to their house. I did like that Teresita's patio gave us a good view of the fireworks being launched from the beach. Teresita serenaded us with the piano. We had a great time.

July 27 brought with it my 26th birthday. My cousins picked me up at my house and took me to my aunt Bobbie's apartment to celebrate. My Godmother Ana Maria, cousins Jeanina, Diana, Lisette and Dino were there. I loved them. I had the greatest birthday time.

In August, I went to San Diego airport and flew to San Francisco. When we arrived, we met up with my grandparents. We had a good time together. On the next day, they went back to Miami. Tia Maricosa and Cousin Junior arrived in San Francisco. We went to the restaurant at the top of the world and sat in our chairs. The restaurant rotated around like Epcot's Universe of Energy ride. It was awesome, and a fantastic view of all of San Francisco.

On the next day, we went inside of the tower to see the view. Then, we went to the science playground at the science center. We had a great time. We went to the pier to catch the ferry to the famous Alcatraz Island. My parents chose not to see it again. Tia Maricosa, Junior and I went to the Alcatraz Prison Museum. It was very interesting. Junior and I stepped into the jail cell for a picture. Inside of my mind, I was acting. I said, *"Help, Mama!"* and *"I need to call my lawyer to get out of jail."* We had fun.

Then, we went back to the ferry and floated back to San Francisco. When we got back, I was glad to see my parents.

On the next day, we went to ride the trolley to the downtown area of San Francisco. We went to the shopping mall. Next we saw Chinatown and the Golden Gate Bridge. We had a great time. We went back to the airport to go home. Tia Maricosa and Junior went back to Miami. They had a great time too.

One evening, I went to Crazy Horse in Costa Mesa by the 55 freeway. We saw Marie Osmond's country performance. I had a great time and I got to shake her hand. I had a great night.

I went back to Miami for Christmas and the New Year. I went to Tia Maricosa's House. My cousins Junior, Mimi and I played "You Don't Know Jack" on Junior's computer. It's a bizarre quiz game with funny commercials and audio. We had great fun.

My grandpa needed help to move his rabbit video transmitter to his bedroom. With this, he could copy video and record his shows.

In the middle of the night, I was sleeping on my grandpa's recliner chair. He went to another recliner and turned on the tv. He was watching a scrambled image and playing only the audio of a channel clearly intended for adults. He had my personality. I was a teenager that liked to watch scrambled pictures and listen to only the audio too. I loved my grandpa Gagan. Then, he went back to bed. I went back to sleep.

After a few days, my mom got a nasty headache and I got a flu and a fever. We had both gotten flu shots before Miami. Gagan, my mom, and my dad took me to the doctor. I got breathing treatments via my grandpa's breathing machine. My mom got better and me too. On Christmas Eve, we celebrated Christmas at Tia Maricosa's house. On Christmas Day, we went to Mark's house in Boca Raton. We had a great Christmas time.

On December 27, we celebrated my dad Norm's birthday with lunch at a restaurant near Mark's jewelry store. We had a great time.

On December 31, we went to Tia Maricosa's house to celebrate the new year of 1997. It was a very good time. I went back home to California on the second day of January.

Chapter Seven:
1997

Mark and Judy came to California to visit me for two days. I had fun with them. I remember we went to the movie theater at Irvine Spectrum and saw the worst movie ever: *The Postman*. Still, we liked Kevin Costner. He played a postman, assigned to deliver the mail. After the movie, my father Norm and Mark were going wild, acting as the postman delivering the mail. My mom, Judy, and I were laughing at them. I loved them. Mark gave us funny nicknames, including me. Mark is the postman. My mom is the pancake maker. My dad is picky (and postman #2). I was 007. I forgot the nickname to call Judy until now. She is a pick penny. We had a fun time.

I went back to Palm Desert for Easter. Everybody met us there. I brought my video game system, a Panasonic 3DO. I invited my family to play Road Rash, a motorcycle racing game. Everybody loved this game. Then we watched a movie in the living room. We had a great time.

We went to Palm Valley clubhouse for Easter brunch. The Easter bunny came, and we took a picture with them. Then we went back home.

I went to my first friend Adam Crow's wedding. I gave him our first picture of us. He loved it. His wedding went great. I had not seen him since I was a kid.

In June, we went back to Miami. My parents had a Cuban Club 25 cruise trip on Destiny. I stayed at my aunt's house. I met a sweet woman called Ahagata, Cousin junior's girlfriend. They were the perfect couple. They took me to the movie theater. I thought it was nice of them to do this.

I went to the cruise ship to say goodbye to my parents and my Mom's friends Berta, Amnery, Mario, Bob, Carmen, and others.

I had a great week without my parents. Cousin Mimi, Cousin Junior and I played "You Don't Know Jack: Volume Two" with hard quizzes and funny commercial ads. Mimi was apparently the smartest of us. We had a great time. Junior had a Tesla ball. I touched it and shocked him. It was funny. I had discovered one of my superpowers.

Seven days later, my parents returned from the cruise. We went back home. I was passed out on the plane ride to California.

I went to the movie theater to see Star Wars's Special Editions. There were hilarious and impressive special effects, and it had the best Dolby Digital surround sound. I saw it twice! I took Sister Debbie and Danielle to see Star Wars: A New Hope.

Jack took me to the movie theater with his grandson Cameron. We saw Disney's Tarzan. I had a bad cough congestion and that made me a bit uncomfortable, but the movie was good. Jack took me home. Afterward.

I think I overdid it thanking him so much.

In October, we went back to Miami for Cousin Mimi's wedding. Before the week of the wedding, my grandparents had the best interview with NBC Nightly News's Bob Dotson about their anniversary. I was there, lurking at the hallway during their interview. It was to be shown on tv later on next summer.

Later, I heard a kitty crying at my grandparents' backyard. Tia Maricosa found it. The poor kitty had gotten lost. I kept the kitty for a few days. The kitty loved me and slept at the outside window.

In the morning, my mom let the kitty inside to the kitchen. She gave the kitty milk and then sent it back outside. I liked to pet the kitty. The kitty gave me a kiss on my cheek. I gave the kitty a chance to sleep on my lap.

My parents said I smelled bad, so I took a bath again. My grandpa picked up the kitty and threw it to the front yard. I was on the other side of the house. Kitty found me, and then kitty went off to another house. I went back to the kitchen to eat my dinner. Guess who showed up at the kitchen window?

The kitty went back to its regular spot at the kitchen window and slept until the next day. I was worrying about the kitty before my Alabama cousins arrived. It was like I knew that these were the last days for us. When they arrived, cousin Manny held the kitty with bad manner. My heart was pounding out of my chest! Cousin John G took the kitty back to its owner at the fourth house. I was sad, and yet I was okay.

One night, all of the cousins (including me) went to the improv comedy club. The show started at 10pm. I don't recall the comedian, but we had a great time. The jokes were funny. At 1:30am, we went back to my grandparents' house to sleep.

We went to the rehearsal for cousin Mimi and Carlos. They had a great practice run for the wedding. Then we went to dinner at the restaurant with the long table. We had a great time.

Everybody came to the church on the wedding day. The wedding went great. I was proud of Mimi and Carlos, a great couple. We went to the reception at the hotel. Mark and Judy came too. I sat at the table with them. Later on, all of the family (grandparents, cousins, uncles, aunts, my parents and I) took a great picture. The wedding went very well.

Then, we danced! I danced with the bride. I was happy. Then, we went outside to say goodbye to the bride and the groom.

A few days later, my parents and I went to see my grandma Vera, aunt Connie and uncle Alex. We went to the beach in Fort Lauderdale. Grandma Vera told me about her life's story. She told about my dad; He was the kind of kid to check the chimney for Santa. She told me lots about her childhood too: looking at the lightbulb for the first time and riding on the train in Virginia as a kid. I enjoyed her stories. When we took her back home, I gave my grandma Vera a kiss on the cheek. We had a great time together.

Someday afterward, we went back home to California. I had a great time in Florida.

Guess who came to California for Christmas and New Year? Our Michigan Family! Sister Linda, Elizabeth, Justin, Jessica and my brother-in-law Don came. We had a great Christmas time. Everybody came here to celebrate one of the best Christmases ever. We took some great family pictures. I wore my best sweater by Tommy Hilfiger. Erika wanted my sweater so much, but I told her no. It's mine. We had a great Christmas time.

The next day, we went to see the Rose Bowl stadium for the first time. We went inside and took a few pictures. We loved it. I saw the word "Michigan" at the touchdown zone on the field. Then we walked Hollywood Boulevard before going home.

That Saturday, we went to Palm Desert. There was heavy traffic on that drive. It took three hours before we arrived at my desert house. That night, we went to the clubhouse for dinner for my father's birthday. We celebrated with Judy, Jack and Marge. We had a fantastic time.

We went to the Marriott hotel to meet my niece Michelle Boyajian from Michigan. Then we went to go shopping at the outlets, one hour away from the desert. My family bought clothing and shoes. It felt good to spend time together.

We went back to our desert home. My parents and Linda and Don went to a New Year's Party at the clubhouse. I stayed with my nieces Elizabeth and Jessica and my nephew Justin. We watched MTV's top 40 music videos and "Dick Clark's Rockin New Year" on ABC broadcast from Time Square in New York.

At 9pm, Justin got a pot and a big spoon. He went outside to bang the pot. I was embarrassed. We waited at midnight, and sure enough Justin banged the pot again. Then my parents, Linda and Don returned from the party and we all went to sleep.

Chapter Eight:
1998

When the first day of the new year was up, we went back to our home in Irvine. On the next day, I went to John Wayne Airport to say goodbye to my sister Linda, Don, Elizabeth, Justin and Jessica- but not before meeting Michigan's football team who had just played in the rose bowl. They all went back to Michigan.

Mark and Judy came back to California. We went to the movie theater and saw the best movie ever: *Titanic*. We enjoyed it. As we left the theater, my dad and Mark acted like characters from the movie. We all laughed. They always kept us joyful.

I went to see Celine Dion in concert at Honda Center. I invited my sister Debbie, Danielle and Tom to join. They came to the concert, but they sat in another section. My dad, my mom and I were in a special section. The stage was at the center of the arena. Celine sang with the Bee Gees and Barbara Streisand on the video screen. She sang "Beauty and the Beast". It was my favorite song that she performed. To conclude, she sang a film song from *Titanic*, "My Heart Will Go On." It was a great show.

We went to Palm Desert on the Wednesday before Easter. That Friday, Gary's family came. My mom and I went to Costco, and while we were there, she told me that my grandpa Gagan was in the hospital. We came back to the desert house with the bad news. I dropped my video games off there for my nieces and nephew to play in my absence. My dad, my mom and I left the desert house to go back to Irvine. I was crying, because my grandpa was dying.

When we got home, we had dinner and packed our suitcases. A limousine arrived and took us to LAX, and we flew to Miami. During the flight, I found that I couldn't sleep. I usually slept on airplanes. When we arrived in Miami we went directly to the hospital and I saw my grandpa. We went to the waiting room and my grand aunt Bobbie was there. Then we went to the cafeteria for breakfast before returning to the room. I was too tired to sit up, so I took a nap in the chair. When I woke up, I had to say farewell to my Grandpa. We left the room. My grandpa was gone. I was very sad. We regrouped at my grandma's house.

On the night of Easter, my luck was low. My mom accidentally shaved a little hair from my forehead. We went to the funeral home and everybody met us there. I was imagining my grandpa Gagan's memories. I loved him and missed him.

On the next day, we went back to the funeral home for mass and to leave my grandpa's body in his resting place. This experience was too emotional. I knew then that I would always miss my best grandpa ever, and his voice as he called to me: "Monkey Boy."

On the next day, my dad flew home to go back to work. My mom and I stayed with my grandma for a week before returning to California. Our cleaner Rosa was crying for us. My dad had told her about us, but Rosa had been confused. She told us that she'd thought we had died. My mom told her about her dad passing away.

I went back to college for P.E., but I did not go inside. I was too depressed about my grandpa's passing. I went to watch the squirrel and the rabbit at the orange trees. Then I went home.

In June, I went to my niece Danielle's 8th grade graduation. She would be going on to high school in the fall. She got her diploma and then we went home.

In the summer, we went to see Danielle's cheerleading performance at Magic Mountain. My mom and I sat in a special section. My family sat up near the top. I was sitting next to a celebrity from *The Young and The Restless*, a popular daytime soap opera. He shook my hand. His name is Kristoff St. John. He was the host of the performance. Danielle's performance went ok. She fell down during her routine, but she was ok. Her team didn't win. However, I had fun at Magic Mountain, so at least someone from our family won that day.

In July, I went to my niece Michelle and her fiancée Mike's fairy tale wedding. The ceremony looked like something out of Cinderella. I enjoyed seeing them together. I had a great time.

On the next day, my dad had 5x bypass open-heart surgery, a week before Erika and Kevin's wedding. He did not go to their wedding. He stayed home with his buddy Jack. My Mom, Totica, Marge, and I went to their wedding. The venue was beautiful. It had a view of a lovely lake in Laguna Niguel. The wedding went great.

My brother Gary went to retrieve my mom's car. He did not return for half an hour. He had broken my mom's car key. He was sweating. My mom said it was ok. Amnery and Mario took us home. Four people filled the back seat. I sat on my mom's lap. On the next day, Gary gave my mom a lift to her car. She had brought another key so that she could bring her car back home.

In August, my 3 nieces (Danielle, Brittney and Lindsay) spent a week with me. We took my scooter to the tunnel. Then they watched *Jerry Springer*. I hated that show. It often displayed people acting as dirty, rowdy lovers that fought each other. It was kind of similar to *Bachelor in Paradise*. The audience said, "Jerry, Jerry, Jerry." It was the most annoying and trashy show ever.

Late at night, just before we went to bed, one of my nieces couldn't sleep, so we watched *The Flinstones* or *Scooby-Doo*. Then, she went back to sleep.

We went to the San Diego Wild Animal Park the next day. It was very hot. We rode the tram to see the animals. My dad held up well despite having a surgery two weeks prior. We had a good time at the park. Late in the night, my nieces couldn't sleep again. They came in my room and we watched The Flinstones or Scooby Doo. Then we went to sleep. It was the first sleepover in my bedroom.

In the middle of August, my cousin told me that my grandparents' video was going to be shown on NBC's Nightly News with Tom Brokaw. I tuned in, but they did not show the video. The next day, I called NBC studios by my relay operator. I gave them a voice message on their answering machine. I also sent them an email.

In the end of August, I got an email from NBC Nightly News. They were going to show my grandparents' video on NBC Nightly News with Tom Brokaw on Friday evening. I became very excited.

But my parents were out of town with Jack and Marge in Arizona. I was staying with Totica. I recorded it on my VCR and showed it to my parents later.

In September, Tia Maricosa and Cousin Junior came back to California. We went to The Getty Museum in Los Angeles. We took a few pictures while we were there. We enjoyed the museum. A few days later, we went to Sony Pictures Studios. We made our way to the studio and waited to be seated in the audience seats. The show was beginning. We were on Donny and Marie. The camera was aimed at us, and you could see my Mom and my Dad, but my shirt was all that could be seen of me on the tv.

We saw Little Richard. He walked slowly to the chair, yet he had a great interview, and played the piano impressively. He sang "Tutti Frutti." Donny Osmond shook my parents hand, but not mine. It's okay, though. The episode was to air in October. After we left the studio, we went to a restaurant in Malibu for dinner. We had a great time.

We took the ferry to Catalina Island. We took a bus tour to the island's little airport and the museum. Then we ate lunch at a restaurant. We went shopping and then we went back to the ferry to go back to Newport Beach. On the next day, we went to Disneyland. We rode a few rides and watched the parade. We had a great time. On the weekend, we went to see Jack's car at the car show. He had a love bug "Herbie" (like the Disney picture.) Jack let me sit in his car and we took a few pictures. I loved old cars.

In December, I went back to Miami for Christmas. I stayed at my grandma Mamama's house. She had a pet. There were yellow canary birds in the kitchen. I slept on my grandpa's recliner chair. Every day, early in the morning around 6:30am, I'd wake up to the birds singing. I tried to go back to sleep, but I could not.

My grandma had a nice maid. She took my Grandma to church in the morning. I missed my Grandpa so much.

On Christmas Eve, we went to Carolina's house. Carolina is Carlos's sister. We had a great time. Then, we went to Espy's mom's house to celebrate Christmas with them. They are my grandpa's brother's family. His brother (Pedro Diaz) called me John Travolta. I saw my cousins. After midnight, we went back to grandma's house. On Christmas Day, we went to Mark's house to celebrate Christmas with my father's family. We had a great time.

Chapter Nine:
1999 and last years of 90s

I went to Palm Desert for the weekend. Mark and Judy drove from Las Vegas to Palm Desert to spend the weekend with me. We went to Palm Springs to go shopping. Before we left Palm Springs, we rode the tram all the way up to the top. It got colder the higher we got, and we were freezing by the time we got to the top. We saw a wonderful view of the Desert. We went back to the club and played some golf. I rode in the golf cart, and even got to take some turns driving. We had a great time. We went back to Irvine and then went to a restaurant in Laguna Beach. A seagull popped up behind Mark, but we didn't feed it. The seagull said, "*Mine, mine, mine..!*" It reminded me of the movie 'Finding Nemo'. This was the last stop in our adventure. Mark and Judy went back to Florida.

In March, I went back to Las Vegas to meet up with Mark and Judy. I stayed at the Hannah hotel. Mark and Judy were staying at The Venetian. They met me at my hotel room and then we walked to their hotel. Judy found some coins on the floor and picked them up. I thought she was lucky to find coins anywhere in Las Vegas. We kept on to their hotel room. I was impressed when I saw it. Their hotel room was outstanding, with a fantastic bathroom to boot. We went to Bellagio for dinner.

On the next day, we went to ride the monorail from Excalibur to New York New York hotel. Then we went to Paris hotel to go inside of the tower. We had a great view of Las Vegas.

We went to Mandalay Bay and had a great lunch. Mark wanted me to play the crap table. I played and I won $70! This was my first win in Las Vegas. After my win, we went back to my hotel room.

My cousins Johnny and Ivette picked me up. We went to Treasure Island hotel to see the pirate show and fireworks. Afterward, they took me back to the hotel. I had a great time with my cousins. That Friday, my parents and I went back to California.

In May, my parents and I went back to Miami. My parents packed suitcases with my grandma Mamama. They were going to drop Mamama off in London so that she could catch a train to Scotland. She was to meet up with her brother Willie and see his family's house. I was staying at my Tia Maricosa's house in Miami for a week. My parents went to Paris while Mamama was in Scotland. They picked Mamama up in London upon her return and brought her back to Florida. I had a great time with my aunt and cousins. My cousin Junior took me to movies. We enjoyed the shows with his buddies and Ahagata. We saw the worst movie ever *Notting Hill.* My parents and Grandma Mamama returned to Florida on a Sunday. They had an adventure of a time.

I went back to my grandma Mamama's house. It was too cold at Tia Maricosa's house. I felt like I had been living in Alaska. My parents and I went to Boca Raton to see Mark's house and visit with my dad's family. We had a great time. Then we went back to California.

On July 4, we went back to Teresita's house in Laguna Beach and watched the fireworks that launched from the beach. We also celebrated Teresita's birthday. We had an awesome time.

In August, I had Brittney and Danielle visit with me for a week. I went to the tunnel and dropped a few pennies there. I went back home and got my nieces. We all went to the tunnel and I challenged them to find the pennies. We had some great fun.

In the evening, I took them to an *NSYNC Concert in Irvine Meadows. I saw Jordan Knight from New Kids on the Block. He performed his solo song before *NSYNC came on. It was good. We had a fun-filled and eventful night. The music was super loud, and my mom had cottons for our ears. We enjoyed the *NSYNC Concert. We left at 11 pm. We went to Carl's JR's drive thru at midnight. We got home and ate a late dinner. Then we went to sleep.

In the fall, my Grandma Mamama came to California to visit with me. We went to Palm Desert that weekend. On Sunday, we went to church and sat in the front row. In the middle of mass, I saw my dad make a mistake and instantly felt sorry for him.

He had gotten the wrong money from the wrong pocket to put in the offering basket. We saw this and we quietly laughed. My poor dad. He did not return his money.

Throughout the 90s, some stores and internet services closed forever.

Gemco (Before Target)

Sav-On (Before CVS)

Alpha Beta (market)

Thrifty (before Rite Aid)

Mayco (before Bloomingdale)

Egghead, the computer store and video game store

Sam Goody Music, Tower Records, and Wherehouse (the place to go for records, cassettes, CDs, videotapes, laserdiscs and music sheets for learning to play.)

Some movie theaters closed

Fedco (before Target)

BBS and Prodigy (internet service providers)

On December 31, I watched and recorded the live 24-hour broadcast of ABC News celebrating the new Millennium: the year 2000 (for the first time in our history.) The Y2K computer virus crashes didn't happen, like a lot of people thought they would. First place was awarded to Tonga: the first country to celebrate the year 2000 at 1am pst.

In either 1997 or 1998, my cousin Mel-Marie came to California. We gave her a tour of stardom, from Beverly Hills to Hollywood to Downtown L.A. We drove to the red carpet of the Oscars. I saw lots of limousines and lots of traffic. I did not see any celebrities. We went home and watched the Oscars on tv. Billy Crystal was the best host of the Oscars ever.

I forgot one thing about Rosa, the lady who cleaned for us: I loved to hide in the closet and scare her while she was vacuuming. We would both laugh. Rosa got married to David at the courthouse. My mom and I were there.

Then we went to Las Brisas restaurant in Laguna Beach. My mom told me, "Why you don't marry her?" I told my mom, "I don't know. She isn't my type."

I got emails from some of my friends from Carl Harvey School- Melissa, Doug, Ryan, Jim, Julie, Alex, Yoalmo and my teachers Mrs. Charbonneau and Mrs. Dunn. it was nice to hear from them.

It's the end of the 1990s.

Chapter Ten:
The year 2000, the 21st century, the new Millennium

I went to my niece Lindsay's concert. She played the violin. She played "The Fate of The Duel" from Star Wars: The Phantom Menace. She did good, and she played well. I enjoyed the concert. I wished that I was a music conductor.

In July, we went back to Fort Lauderdale for Grandma Vera's 100th birthday. We stayed in a special condominium by the beach. Everybody came from everywhere- from Michigan, California and Maryland. Before party day, we went to the market with my sister Linda and got a few groceries. At the cashier, Betty made a bad comment about my nephew Justin to my mom. My mom grew angry, and I could tell by the way that she responded. Betty apologized to my mom. We went back to the condominium and had a pool party. Tia Maricosa and Gary played tabletop ping pong. Everybody came to this pre-party party. We had a great time.

At 7am the next day, we walked out to the beach. My sister Linda wanted me to go into the ocean. She helped me take off my shoes and we walked to the water. It was very cold. I went back to my chair. Afterwards, we got ready for the biggest party ever.

We went to the place where the party was going to be held and waited for the party room at the second level to be available. As we entered the party room, my sister Debbie looked to the video camera and said, "Hello, I am Debbie from California!" I think that we had about 200 people present.

I sat with my nephew Justin, my nieces Jessica and Elizabeth, and Erika and Kevin. We ate our lunch together.

Then, we danced to funk and conga music. We had a ball. Grandma Vera got a special gift, a signed shirt from Oprah. We sang happy birthday to her. Then, we all took pictures with Grandma Vera. We had the greatest birthday party ever. Then, we went back to the condo and I was met with a surprise: Mark had got a special 007 birthday cake for my early 30th birthday. I laughed, and I smiled as they sang happy birthday to me.

The next day, we drove to Orlando for my birthday trip with family, including Jack and Marge. I rode in a van with Jack, Marge and Tia Maricosa. My parents and family were in another van. We drove for four hours and only made one rest stop. We arrived in Orlando and my mom got the keys to the rental house. It had a pool and 4 bedrooms.

On the next day, we went to Epcot for the whole day. We went on the Spaceship Earth, Into the Imagination, The Living Seas (the aquarium), Universe of Energy with Ellen DeGeneres on screen (and an animated Ellen with a dinosaur), The Land, and a few countries. We had dinner at the French restaurant in

(Epcot's) Paris. Then we watched the parade and fireworks by the lake. We enjoyed this park. We went back to the house.

On the next day, we went to Disney's Studio. We went to the animation studio to see how the next animated films would work. Then, we went on the trams, sort of like the type for the universal studios tour. We had lunch at the restaurant near the "Honey, I Shirked the Kids" playground.

We went to Muppets 4D and had fun. Tia Maricosa took Nana to the restroom. But when my Tia checked, she was not there. Nana was outside. Tia Maricosa found her and got a wheelchair for her. We didn't want to lose her again. At the end of the day, we went back to the house.

On the next day, everybody went to the pool at the backyard. Sean, Phil and Mark came up to the house. They were very nice cousins. In the evening, we went to the House of Blues at Downtown Disney.

We sat down at the long table, close to the stage where the musician played. We celebrated my birthday again because some of us were leaving tomorrow. Sean, Mark and Phil went back to Boca Raton.

On the next day, Tia Maricosa, my mom and I went to Walt Disney World. We rode the PeopleMover and Winnie the Pooh rides. I loved this ride. During the Tigger scene, the ride bounced around crazily. We went back to the house and I babysat Baby Marlena. She looked at me and smiled. I was glad. Everyone else went to have fun at Walt Disney World.

Linda, Don, Elizabeth, Justin and Jessica came for their last visit before they went back to Michigan. We took a few pictures to cherish our moments. Some of our family went back to California. Cousin Junior and Ahagata came to Orlando. Also, Cousin Yuyi, Eric and Jason came. Junior, Eric, Jason and I went to the movie theater. We saw the first X-Men movie. We enjoyed it. We went back to the house. I had a great birthday.

On the next day, my parents, Jack, Marge and I went to Orlando Airport to go back to California, our home sweet home.

OCTA needed me to re-register at the office in Anaheim. The bus picked my mom and I up at my house. We went to the office and waited for a half hour for my turn. I re-registered for bus transportation services. We hated waiting afterwards for the bus to take us home at 4pm. We'd had no lunch, so we were even more pissed. It was the worst transport ever, in decades. Now my mom wanted to help me throw the bus into the ocean.

In September, my parents and I went to Miami for cousin Junior and Ahagata's wedding. We stayed at my grandma Mamama's house. She had got an ugly old pug named Alejo. He loved to sleep.

On the big night, I went to see Cousin Junior and Ahagata's wedding at their church. They got married and we all went to the reception. I had a great time at the reception. I danced with many people, including the bride, the gorgeous ladies, my mom, and my aunt. We had a great night.

A few days later, we took Mamama and Alejo to California for two weeks. Alejo was in a bag at the airport. As we rode the elevator, Alejo's head popped out and scared the airport security. We all laughed. We boarded the plane and flew to California.

In the morning, my mom and I were eating our breakfast. Alejo came to the kitchen and sat down by my mom. She gave Alejo a slice of cheese. He loved it. We had one small problem: Alejo peed at the wood table in the living room! My dad put caution tape at the living room columns.

Sometimes, Alejo would come to my room and take a nap. I'd be watching tv. Then he'd go back to Mamama. I had to look after Alejo one night. I opened the sliding door for him when he needed to pee. He'd waddle right back inside when he was done.

One day, Alejo and I were at the front hallway. He started barking at the mailman, so I held him back. He was ferocious.

On their last day in California, I took Mamama and Alejo to the airport and they went back to Miami.

I went to Danielle's play at her high school. She was a great actress. I liked the play. I wanted to go back to my college and take an acting class sometime in the future. I didn't want to do it alone though.

On New Year's Eve, we celebrated my father Norm's 70th birthday party ever. I recorded video of the party and made my first live video stream to the internet from a wireless camera. I also gave my dad the best present ever. It was a picture puzzle!

Cousins Mark, Judy and Phil came to California for my father's 70th birthday. We had a big tent in my backyard. The weather was very cold. I had bought some confetti, a few party horns and some New Year hats for the evening. Everybody you could think of came to this party. We had a great time together. I was chatting with family and friends who were only able to attend via the internet. We celebrated by giving my dad a birthday cake. Before midnight, everybody went inside to watch Dick Clark's Rockin New Year's Eve countdown until the ball dropped from Time Square in New York.

Everybody got some pop confetti. We were excited for midnight to come.

10… 9… 8… 7… 6… 5… 4… 3… 2… 1…

Chapter Eleven:
2001

10, 9, 8, 7, 6, 5, 4, 3, 2, 1- Happy New Year! Everybody popped the confetti into the air. This wasn't well planned- we made a huge, glittery mess of things. We had fun though. We turned the music loud and danced. 20 minutes later, the cops came to ask us to turn it down. I had forgotten to turn off the outside speakers. Everybody left my house around 1:30 am. We cleaned up the confetti with our vacuum and with a broom and a trash bag. Mark, Judy and Phil helped us out. They spent the night at my house. We were too tired to go to the Rose Parade in the morning. We hadn't gotten to sleep until 3 am.

That afternoon, Mark, Judy and Phil took me as their GPS to Dana Point and Laguna Beach, and through the uphill roads to see the houses in Laguna Beach. The road was dangerous. I felt scared. It was like riding a roller coaster. We took a walk through the shops in Laguna Beach before heading home.

On the next day, we went to the Beverly Hills Hotel to have a look inside at the Golden Globes award stage. Then we went to Rodeo Drive to walk the shops and had lunch at the McCormick & Schmick's restaurant. My mom wanted me to pay for everyone's lunch with my MasterCard. I was shocked and embarrassed at them. Still, I paid. Mark took a picture of me signing my bill and another picture of all of us together. We had a great day. After dinner, we went back home.

That night, I thought it would be funny to create my own shopping channel and use my wireless camera to transfer the video to the tv screen in the den. I acted like I was selling my shoes for $99. I had made a sign for the big sale. My channel looked like QVC, or the home shopping network. I heard my family laughing very hard from the den.

On the next day, Mark and Judy would leave to go back to Florida and Phil would head back to Maryland. I had a lot of fun with them.

On January 30, my parents went to Laguna Beach Hospital before the sun had come up. My niece Erika was trying to deliver her baby boy. I was asleep in my bed. When my parents got back, Erika was still in the hospital. No baby had come yet.

January 30 was my mom's birthday too. She was excited to have her grandchild.

Late in the morning, we went to the hospital and sat in the waiting room. Then we went to the cafeteria to have some lunch. Then we went back to the waiting room. Around 2pm, my nephew was born. He is named Tyler. I was glad to have a baby boy in our family. He was a wonderful baby. Everybody came to see my nephew Tyler.

We had to babysit Tyler on weekdays. He was a good baby boy. My mom gave him his milk and played a Spanish Lullaby cd to put him to sleep. He would wake up and smile at me. He enjoyed his swing chair. Tyler made me happy. I thought he was a funny baby. I had fun with him.

We went back to Palm Desert for our last Easter weekend in the desert house. Everybody came to join us. We had great fun, and we also celebrated Nana's birthday. It was the last time that our whole family would be together.

We went to La Crescenta National Park. I hated the narrow roads wrapping around the mountain. I was very nervous. My mind said, *"I don't want to die!!!"* We finally arrived at Nana's family reunion in La Crescenta National Park. They had a zip lining activity that some people from our family enjoyed. Baby Tyler was in a wagon. Nana spent time with her cousins, and I think that she had a great time. My parents and I went back home safely. We did not die on the mountain.

In May, we had Marlena's first birthday party ever at my house. Alicia shot a video. Everybody came, including Amnery, Rosa, Brittany, and Josefina. We had a great time. On the next day, we went to the pool. I drove my scooter there. After the pool, my mom walked home with me. When we got to our street, my mom did the worst thing ever to my scooter: She took off the break. I was very scared, and I was reminded just how much I did not want to die! The scooter went super-fast on its way downhill.

I yelled, "Help!!" Mike was packing a suitcase in his truck. My mom yelled for him, "Mike!" He asked me, "Do you need help?" I nodded my head yes. He ran and saved both me and my scooter. I gave him thanks for saving me. I was very upset with my mom.

In June, Jessica and Linda came to California for a week. Cyndee would come later, bringing Brittney along. We went to the new Disney's California Adventure for the first time. It was different from Disneyland and had roller coasters. The girls went on the rides. We watched the electric parade together. We got home at midnight.

The next day, we went to Palm Desert. My dad said, "I need oxygen." It was very hot, so we went to the pool. We had a great time. The next day, we went to the outlets, and then we went back to Irvine.

On the next day, Cyndee came. We took a ride on the electric boat at Balboa Island with Jack and Marge. Jack was the captain. He looked like Captain from The Love Boat.

On July 4, Jack, Marge, my parents, and I went to John Wayne airport and transferred to LAX. We boarded another plane and flew to Vancouver, Canada. It was our first time in Canada. We saw blue fireworks soon after arriving at our hotel. It was like a new sunset, happening at night. Then we walked to a restaurant about a block away from the hotel.

We waited about half an hour for our dinner to be served. Canada took a long time to cook dinner. Afterwards, we walked back to the hotel.

On the next day, we went to the Classical Chinese Garden Museum. It's a special museum in Canada. I took a video. We enjoyed it. Then, we went to Downtown Vancouver for lunch. We saw a musical clock whistling with smoke. We liked it. My dad told Jack that he had to get one. Then we took a bus tour of all the cities of Vancouver. The driver was very talkative about Vancouver.

After a few stops in different places, Jack, my dad and I stayed inside the bus for the rest of the tour. We did enjoy the tour though. We went back to the hotel when it was done.

On the next day, we got on the ferry with our red rental van and went to Victoria Island. We had a breakfast on the ferry. The trip took two hours.

When we got to Victoria Island, we went to The Butchart Gardens. The guys did not go inside. I went in with my mom and Marge. The garden was spectacular and featured a fountain show. I felt like I was in *Alice in Wonderland*. We enjoyed it. Two hours later, we went back to the van and returned to the ferry.

Two hours later, we were back in Vancouver. We went to the shopping mall. It had three levels of stores. It was different from American malls. We had a great time.

On the next day, we drove to Whittler mountain. This took two hours and thirty minutes. It was snowy, and darn cold on Whittler mountain. We got a rental condominium with a beautiful view of Snow mountain. I watched KTLA 5 from Canada's cable television. I hated that the sunrise came at 4:00 am. It was too early.

On the next day, we went to play golf. I took a video. We had fun. The following day, we dropped Jack and my dad off at the golf course. The ladies and I went shopping at the village.

We picked the guys up from the golf course afterwards. They had a great time. We went back to the condominium.

Another day, it was very rainy. The guys couldn't play golf on our last day. We went to the restaurant for lunch. Then we went back to the condominium for rest.

On the next day, we drove back to Vancouver through heavy traffic. It took three hours. When we arrived in Vancouver we went to a restaurant for lunch. I did not know that this restaurant had a handicap restroom on the ground floor. Next, we went shopping at Downtown Vancouver. I bought a Davy Crockett hat. We had a great time.

We got a comfy suite for our last day in Canada. On the next day, we went to the airport and headed home to California. We had a great time in Canada.

I had missed my nephew Tyler for a week. I could tell that he had missed us too. I took a picture of Tyler in my Canada hat.

On July 16, I went to see Jurassic Park 3 by myself. My parents went to see another movie with Jack and Marge. I entered into the darkness. I was walking down the aisle and I saw a guy with glasses, but he did not see me, and he bumped into me. I fell down and hurt my right hand. The guy said, "Sorry." He helped me up and I went to my seat. After the movie, I went home and went to the bathroom. I yelled "Mama!!!" I had broken my right ring finger.

A few days later, I went to my doctor to get a brace for my finger. It took a few months to get it back straight. It was painful.

In August, my grandma Mamama and Alejo returned to California to visit with us for two weeks. We had a great time. Then they went back to Miami.

On August 28, Rosa had a baby girl. My mom and I went to the hospital and saw a beautiful baby girl. She is named Brittany Danielle Clary. She grew up and made my first book cover for me. I will tell more of that story in the next book. For now, we gave Rosa congratulations.

In the end of August, I went to Palm Desert for the weekend. Erika and Tyler came. We took a picture of Tyler with his Halloween costume on. He was Dumbo the elephant. He looked very cute. We also celebrated Lindsay's birthday. We had a good time in Palm Desert. I still hated the traffic going home.

On September 11, 2001, I woke up and walked into my parents' bedroom. We saw awful news, a tragic moment in history on tv. We watched an ABC News Special Report. The terrorists had hijacked the planes that crashed into the World Trade Center buildings, into the Pentagon in Washington DC, and into the ground in Philadelphia. We were shocked badly and saw president George W. Bush was in a school in Florida when the secret service told him that America was under attack. We were sad. I am sorry for all of the people who were hurt or lost in the attacks of September 11, 2001.

I went to see Danielle's cheerleading at the high school football game. She did good as a cheerleader. I don't remember who won the football game. Who cares? Afterward, we went to the restaurant for dinner with Danielle. We had some great fun.

On Thanksgiving, we went to Mark's house in Florida, and brought Mamama with us. We celebrated Thanksgiving there. We had a great time. Afterwards, we went back to Mamama's house.

I made a big mistake about my grandma and her house. I saw a huge stack of old mail, past due bills in the drawer. I was worried about that. I told my Alabama Uncle Puncho and Aunt Beba to come and take care of her. I wished I had a time machine to fix this. They took my grandma and moved her away to Alabama. I thought it was my fault that they took my grandma to Alabama, and I considered it to be one of my biggest mistakes ever. I went back to California.

In December, we went back to Miami. We stayed at Tia Maricosa's house. Then, I met my cousin Mimi's first daughter Elisa (Eli) for the first time ever. She was a good baby. I took two videos of Eli. We celebrated Christmas Eve at Tia Maricosa's home. We went to the living room to open the presents. I gave Mimi an internet video camera.

On Christmas Day, we went to Paul's house to celebrate Christmas with my dad's family. We had a great time and opened even more presents.

On New Year's Eve, my parents and I went to Mark's house to see my father's family, including Phil's family. I met Mark and Judy's dog, Penny. She was a good, loving dog. We slept at Mark's house. Penny climbed onto my bed early in the morning, before Mark went to work at his jewelry shop. Later, we celebrated our New Year's Eve party, and Grandma Vera's 102nd birthday at Mark's house. We went to watch tv, for Fox News' countdown to 2002.

Everybody yelled, "*10... 9... 8... 7... 6... 5... 4... 3... 2... 1...*"

Chapter Twelve:
2002

10...9...8...7...6...5...4...3...2...1... Happy New Year!!!!!! We sang Auld Lang Syne in silly tones of voice. Mark played a cd with some conga music. My family would dance out onto the patio and back into the house, then back to the patio, then back into the house. I shot video of the whole thing. We had a great time. Everybody left around 1:30 am. I went to sleep on the sofa bed.

Early in the morning, Penny jumped on the sofa bed and licked me before jumping back down. Mark came to me and said, "Happy New Year." We had a great breakfast, and then we said our goodbyes. We went back to Miami for our last day in Florida. On the next day, I saw the opening of the Rose Parade on TV. We were ready to go to the airport. We went back to California, our home sweet home.

My parents and I went to see Lindsay's basketball game. She was a very good basketball player. Lindsay's team won, with 35 points over the other team's 15 points. We enjoyed her game.

I went to Tyler's first birthday party. I did not know about the time capsule that was being made for Tyler's 18th birthday. I gave him my big book of Walt Disney's Animation, my little transporter jeep, and a birthday letter. I made him a birthday video and burned it to CD-ROM for his time capsule. I had a great time at the party.

Before I could leave to go home, Tyler started crying. He wanted to go with us.

I went back to Palm Desert for the weekend. Bob and Carmen bought a desert house. Amnery and Mario came and stayed at my Desert house. We had a great time. A few weekends later in Palm Desert, I was driving the golf cart in the Oasis Country Club area. It was very windy, and something of a sandstorm was stirred up. I got sand in my teeth. It made a crunching sound. It tasted awful. I hated this weather.

Back in Irvine, I had Tyler on weekdays again. We went to the park together. We fed bread to the ducks and the geese. We went to the playground. Tyler liked to slide on the slide and swing on the swings. I swung on the swing with him. We had a great time. Some afternoons, we took naps on my bed. I woke up once to Tyler's head on my chest. I whispered to my mom. She was playing a computer game in the office. I whispered to her again. I needed to go to the bathroom. She came and moved him to my bed. I ran to the bathroom. Tyler was still sleeping for another hour. He woke up and smiled.

We went to South Coast Plaza mall, and my dad, Tyler and I went on the carousel. My mom was camera-lady. Then, we went to the Oakley Factory in Foothill Ranch to get my dad's sunglasses. The Oakley Factory looked like a weird empire building from Star Wars.

Inside, I saw a big car with a snake logo on the wall. I went to sit in the old airplane chair. Then we went to see the cannon. It was like a museum.

In March, we went to Maui with Jack and Marge. We got a rental condo in Wailea Gold Golf Club. My parents and Jack and Marge played a few rounds of golf. They had a great game. I rode in the golf cart with my mom and Marge.

Then, we went to Lahaina, Maui for Jack's favorite hamburger restaurant, Cheeseburger in Paradise. The restaurant had an upstairs, and this is where our table was. We had a good time here. Then, we saw a rainbow in Maui. We went back to the condominium and took a video of the sunset.

On the next day, we went to Kapalua Beach, Maui to see the beach and the big waves on the ocean. It was very windy. On the last day, we went to Costco in Maui. It's the same as in California, except the workers where Maui shirts instead. Later into the evening, we went to the airport to go back to California.

We took Tyler to the Irvine Zoo park. He saw the sheep. Erika put the sheep food in Tyler's hand and he almost ate it. She said, "No, it's for the sheep!" He laughed. We saw a few animals at this zoo. He had a great bunch of fun. We went on the train ride and Tyler rode a pony. He laughed. We had a great time.

On April 12, we drove 6 hours to northern California for Alicia's Hawaiian 12th birthday party at Morris's house on April

13. We made one stop at Sweet Pea's soup restaurant for lunch, and then we got back on the freeway, eventually arriving at our hotel.

After stopping by our hotel, we went to Michelle's house with its steep uphill driveway. It was hard to walk uphill to her house. We went inside to see Alicia, Joey and Marlena. We had dinner there. Then, we went back to the hotel to sleep.

On the next day, we went back to Michelle's house, and then drove to Morris' house to celebrate Alicia's birthday party. Joey and Erika were jumping on the giant trampoline in the backyard. They went walking down to the lake. When they came back, Alicia opened her gifts. We sang happy birthday to Alicia. We had a great birthday party thru to the night. When the party was done, we went back to the hotel. On the next day, we drove back home.

Sometime before the spring, Alejo died in Alabama. My grandma Mamama went to a senior home in Mobile, Alabama. In May, I went to Mobile, Alabama for Mother's Day week. I stayed at Tio Puncho and Tia Beba's house. We went to pick up my grandma Mamama from the senior home and took her to their house. We celebrated Mother's Day with all of our Alabama family. We had a good time.

When we woke up the next morning, my parents went to play golf. I stayed at the house with my Aunt Beba and Uncle Puncho and tried to go back to sleep. Beba was a little strange.

She wanted me to get up and walk around the back patio. So, I did.

After a while I went back to the living room and Beba left me be. I felt like something strange was going on. When we left, we took my grandma Mamama back to California to stay with us for a month.

But I ended up keeping my grandma in California. I thought that my grandma would be better off here with us. Two months later, I found a senior home in Irvine. It was only one mile away from our home. Mamama loved it, and I loved that I was able to help her.

Tyler enjoyed playing my dad's harmonica. I took a video of him playing. He also liked to pull his toys from the chest box and bring them out to my patio. He was a good boy.

In June, I went to Danielle's high school graduation. She wore a red gown, just like I did for my Carl Harvey School graduation. She was a beautiful niece. She got a diploma and threw her red hat in the air. We went to her apartment and had cake and saw her gifts. She had one of the greatest graduations ever.

On my 32nd birthday, Amnery, Mario, Carmen, Bob, Mamama, Jack, Marge, Debbie, Danielle, Erika, Tyler, Linda and Justin came to celebrate with me at the patio. I loved this time.

I went to a restaurant in Palm Desert and lost my graduation ring again. This time, I would not find it.

My parents and I were thinking about selling our desert house the next year. We were getting tired of driving to Palm Desert thru more and more traffic and even more people. We went to a new casino in the desert. I played the slot machine, but I had no luck. My mom got lucky and won a little money. I was glad for her. We had a good night.

We brought our swing lounge from the Desert house to our home in Irvine.

Sometimes in the afternoon at home in Irvine, when my dad would come home from his job, he'd go to the kitchen and start to cook some eggs. Then, he would leave the kitchen. He would forget his eggs. I would hear popping sounds coming from the kitchen, and yell, *"Papa!!"* By the time he got them, the eggs were spoiled rotten. He wouldn't even eat the poor eggs. He instead threw them away to the trash.

My parents and Jack and Marge went to Honolulu. I was staying home with Totica. That Saturday afternoon, I was out on the swing when I saw a strange plane. It looked like a stealth plane, or a UFO. I needed Mulder and Scully from The X Files (cue iconic whistle tunes). The plane was moving slowly toward my house. I ran into my room to get my camera, but when I got back, the plane was gone. The sliding door was not working, and I couldn't lock it.

Totica and I were frustrated with the sliding door. It was just one inch away from closing. Totica could not sleep well that night. She got a knife and went to sleep on the couch.

The next day, Totica was coughing and feeling ill. Later into the afternoon, she got worse. I called my mom and told her that Totica was sick and I hadn't taken a bath in two days. At 4am, Rosa knocked on my window. I opened the door. She came in and checked on Totica. Totica was not doing well. Rosa told my mom via the phone. Totica's sister Zelda came and cared for Totica. My parents arrived the next morning. Totica was doing a little better. This was the last time she took care of me.

On Halloween night, I went to Tyler's house to trick or treat. Tyler was Mickey Mouse. We walked just one block to trick or treat. We had a great time.

We celebrated Thanksgiving Dinner at my house. My brother Gary brought his girlfriend Marie for the first time. She was quiet. He had moved on from his past, and he loved Marie now. We had a great time together.

On Christmas Day, we celebrated with dinner at my house again. We had a great meal. Then, we went to the living room to open the Christmas presents.

Poor Tyler took his presents to the den to open them. My mom told him that it was the twilight zone. She gave him an electric car for Christmas; But he was too afraid to have fun with it! We kept his car in storage until next Christmas. We had the greatest Christmas ever.

Chapter Thirteen:
2003

In January, Phil, Mark, and Judy came back to California and stayed at my house. We went to President Ronald Reagan's library museum. It's a bigger museum than President Nixon's library museum. It had a few old planes, and we went inside of Reagan's Air Force One. I had a great time, and a long day. We went to a restaurant with Judy C, Marge and Jack. We had a great dinner. On the next day, we went to San Diego's Hotel del Coronado for lunch with Jack and Marge. We had a great time, although I knew there was a ghost there. We drove back home, a 2-hour trip. On the next day, Mark, Judy, and Phil left California to go back to their home.

I took an online chess history class from Irvine Valley College for the first time. I loved it. I got a B grade for this class.

In the spring, Justin and his roommate came to California for the weekend. They stayed at an apartment close to Warner Bros. Studio. My parents and I picked them up, and we went to Santa Monica Pier and downtown Santa Monica. We went to a restaurant for lunch. We had a good time. Then we dropped them back off to the apartment.

In May, I went back to Florida. We stayed at Mark's house for a few days. We went to Fort Lauderdale beach to walk with Connie, Judy, and Liz.

Grandma Vera stayed home alone. She was 103 years old. When we got back to her house, I kissed Grandma Vera's cheek. Then we went to Miami and stayed with Tia Maricosa for a week.

I met Cousin Mimi's second daughter Tessie. She was a good baby girl. I played with Eli with her toy. She smiled at me. Junior and Ahagata and Luz came to Tia Maricosa's house. Junior, Javi and I went to the movie theater to see the second *Lord of The Rings* movie. I thought it was okay, but they loved it. A few days later, we went to back to California.

In June, we went to Brittney's high school graduation in Rancho Cucamonga. I didn't like that we had to look through fences to watch her graduation. It was a good graduation, though. My mom took a video as Brittney got her diploma. She was excited. I was glad to see her graduation.

We went to Brittany's baptism. My mom was named Brittany's godmother. She didn't like having to get wet. She was baptized. Then, we went to her house. She had a DJ at her backyard. We had a good time.

A few days later, we took Tyler to the Santa Ana Zoo. We saw lots of monkeys, peacocks, sheep and pigs. Tyler went to the playground with my dad. They had a great time.

Linda, Elizabeth, and Jessica came back to California. Erika and Tyler met up with us and we went shopping at Rodeo Drive in Beverly Hills. We had a good lunch at a restaurant.

Then, we got back to shopping. I saw a tv reality star for the first time, the guy from Joe Millionaire (another dating show on FOX less like The Bachelor).

Erika asked him to take a picture with her uncle. He answered yes. We took a picture together. Then, we went back home. Tyler and I watched Shrek on the tv in Erika's SUV. We had a good time.

In August, I went to Amnery's luau party at her patio. Little girl Natalia was dancing with the hula girls. She was too cute. Natalia is Amnery's godchild.

I saw a giant cooked pig at the table. It was disgusting to see. My dad took a picture of the pig and my mom. We had a good party, despite the pig.

We went to Cousin Jeanina's wedding. Her husband's name is Hernando, hailing from Argentina and California. He is a great guy for Jeanina. I was so happy for them. I took lots of pictures of the wedding. We had a great time at the reception and enjoyed dancing. I was dancing with my cousins. I got home at eleven that night. Another day, we went to my godmother's house and we saw Jeanina and Hernando opening their wedding presents. I gave them $100. They were very happy together.

In September, we went to Brittany's 2nd birthday party at her house in Corona. She was happy. She had a great entertainer for her birthday party. I took Tyler there. We had a great time.

We went to Disneyland with Tyler, Brittany, Rosa and Josefina. Rosa's son Fernando was working at Disneyland Lights. He gave us our passes. We went inside to Main Street, USA. We saw Minnie Mouse. We took a picture of she and I. I heard Minnie's kissing sound and she gave me a kiss on my cheek.

I was wondering if Mickey would get jealous about it. Then we went to Frontierland to the Winnie the Pooh ride. But it is not the same as the version at Walt Disney World. It doesn't have the bounce in the ride for the Tigger scene, and it was different from the other park. Brittany and Tyler took a few pictures of Eeyore, Tigger and Pooh.

We went to Fantasyland, where we rode on Dumbo, the flying elephant. Then, we went to the *It's a Small World* ride and enjoyed it twice. Then we went to Toontown. We rode the Roger Rabbit ride. We went to the toon jail to take a picture of us. Next, we went to the toon car to take pictures of Brittany and Tyler. We saw real ducks in the grass in Fantasyland and at Main Street. Tyler fed them popcorn, and then we went back to Main Street for the parade. The kids got cotton candy. We watched the parade before leaving and heading home.

A few days later, my grandma Mamama's friend Kiki died. We went to her funeral. But I did not know that they would do a double funeral service: one in English and one in Spanish. It took 3 hours. We hadn't had lunch yet and the weather was very hot. We made it thru and left to go back home.

Someday soon after, my parents went to play golf. I got a cooler, my lunch and a water bottle, plus some napkins. I put my cooler on my scooter, pulled it out, got on and closed the garage door. I was riding my scooter to see my grandma 1½ mile away and took 25-30 minutes. I felt like little red riding hood on my way to Grandma's house. I arrived at my grandma's senior home. She was so happy to see me. She had already eaten lunch.

Still, my grandma liked to go and sit in the cafeteria. We gave my lunch to a server. She cooked my lunch and returned it to me, and then I ate my lunch. When I was done, we went back to my grandma's room. I stayed for an hour. Then, I went back home. I got home safe, with no big bad wolf.

My grandma got a scooter. But she bumped the elevator and ran over somebody's foot. She was speeding too fast. Wait until you hear what happened to me on Halloween.

Mamama, my mom and I went to see the tv talk show *Beyond with James Van Praagh,* live in person. James is a medium who talks with dead people. They were filming double episodes at KTLA 5's studios in Hollywood. We waited for a few hours after our arrival to go inside the studio. I was super happy that I would be shown on tv, and double episodes at that!!

We didn't get to hear anything from my grandfather Gagan. James said, "Picky." My mom was shocked- but it was for a lady below us, a message from her dad. The light bulb went out during the second episode. I wanted to copy these episodes with our special cameos on videotape or DVD very badly.

After we left the filming, we went to eat a late lunch and dinner at Old Spaghetti Factory in Hollywood. We hadn't had lunch before the show. We went back home.

On Halloween, I went to my grandma Mamama's senior home. I entered her room. I was waiting for her to get ready to go to her Halloween parade and party downstairs. She wore a mafia mask with a fake cigar. I walked out to the hallway while filming a video. She roared out of her room on her scooter. She ran into me in the hallway and I fell down with my video camera. My mom asked her if she could see through her mask. I was ok. We went to the elevator and Mamama banged into it with her scooter. She was dangerous with her mask on. At least, we wanted to say that it was because of the mask.

We went to the party and parade with her friends Lilly and France. I took a few videos of the party. We had a great time.

Then, my parents and I went to Erika's house for Tyler's trick or treat. Tyler was Tigger. Erika was Winnie the Pooh. Kevin was hip-hop Kaptain Gangster. I was wearing a cap with muffler hair. My mom was a Chinese lady and my dad was rock star Ozzy Osbourne with black hair and black eye makeup. We went out to trick or treat with Tyler. We had a good time.

In December, Junior, Ahagata and Luz came to California for our grandma Mamama's 86th birthday. We all celebrated together. The next day, we went to the park with Tyler and fed the ducks and geese.

Then we went to the playground. We had a great time, but I turned out with a bad cough. We went home. Rosa, Josefina and Brittany came to visit us. I did not feel good. I went to sleep on my bed. Another day, I went to my doctor and got prescribed antibiotics. I took a few naps. At night, Ahagata spent time with me for their last day in town. They were leaving back to Miami.

On New Year's Eve, we went to Pasadena. Elizabeth and her friend were at the motel. We picked them up to get lunch at some restaurant in Pasadena. They were going to the Rose Bowl game for Michigan's team (Go Blue!). After lunch, we took them back to the motel. We gave them a goodbye and a Happy New Year.

Later on, my parents went to a party. I was home alone. I watched "Dick Clark's Rockin' New Year" countdown to 2004.

Chapter Fourteen:
2004

We went to Laguna Beach with Erika and Tyler for a special photoshoot. Erika was the photographer. My mom held a light shade for the photoshoot. We had a good time.

I went to Tyler's 3rd birthday bash at Irvine Park. They have a train ride there. Tyler was dressed as a train conductor. We all took a trip on the train ride, and we enjoyed it. After the ride, we sang happy birthday to Tyler. Then we regrouped at his house to open his presents. My dad, my mom and I gave him a guitar. He spent some time playing it and singing his smash hit "*Oh*." He had a great birthday.

We went to the hospital to see my new nephew Mason, the son of Gary and Marie. He was a small baby boy. Everybody in our family came to see him.

Two weeks later, we went back to the same hospital to see my new second-generation nephew Garrett, the son of niece Brittney and Rob. Garrett was a special baby boy. Mason is Garrett's uncle! It was a pretty cool event in our family.

Cousin Junior came to California for his work in Los Angeles for the weekend. He was on TV, featured in the Spanish news program. He came back to Irvine by way of the train. Together, we visited our grandma Mamama.

Then, Sunday afternoon, we went to see a house tour in Newport. Junior tried to scare my Mom…but he accidentally scared the wrong person. He was very embarrassed. I laughed at my cousin. Later, Junior went back to LA, again by way of the train. A while later, he went back to Florida.

My grandma Mamama got a hobby. She started painting at her senior home. She painted pretty well, too. She liked it. She made a painting of a horse and country scenery. She had my Mom's painting personality.

I went to NASA's Jet Propulsion Laboratory (JPL) in Los Angeles with Joey, Tyler, and Debbie. I think Joey made a robot fighter, but I am honestly not quite sure if that's what it was. The weather was very hot. There were too many people there, so many people that it felt like a zoo of humans. Still, we had a good time.

Erika, Tyler, my mom, and I went to see *Sesame Street* live in Hollywood at the Dolby Theatre. Rosa, Brittany, and Josefina were there also. I remembered that when I was a kid, my mom took me to see *Sesame Street on Ice* in Long Beach. We enjoyed that show back then, and we enjoyed this production in Hollywood now.

Then, we went to see the giant tv screen displaying the filming of *On the Air with Ryan Seacrest*, a talk show. I saw his studio through the window. We ate lunch at a restaurant. We had a great time in Hollywood.

One day, my mom, Tyler and I went outside, and my mom took a few pictures of the two of us. Tyler was posing like me. My mom laughed and took a picture. Tyler was a very funny kid.

I went back to Miami Beach, where I stayed at a condominium near the shore. On Memorial Day, we went to the beach. My cousins came and joined us. We had the greatest Memorial Day ever.

Later in the night, Luz Cristina was up on the kitchen table and it broke down under her. It was an accident. My mom and Tia Maricosa bought another table to replace it.

I went to Mimi's house and played with Tessie. She was playing with her teacup with me. I noticed that Mimi started tearing up at her eyes. She had become emotional, in a good way. We had a good dinner. We played the continental card game. My dad took his sweet time on each of his turns. We were all waiting for him impatiently. I had a great time.

We picked up Sister Debbie at the airport. She stayed with us. We went to Brad and Liz's wedding place on the weekend. Everybody came there. Even Grandma Vera was there at 104 years old (though she was in a wheelchair). Mark, Phil, Connie, and Judy visited in my room.

Then, we went to the rehearsal dinner and watched the tribute video full of Brad and Liz's pictures. They were crying. They loved it. I met Alfred's wife Lori and her son Chase. But Alfred had died of a heart attack. I met him back at Grandma Vera's 95th and 100th birthday parties.

On the wedding day, we got ready for Brad and Liz's wedding. It was outside with a view of the ocean. I sat down with my sister Debbie. The wedding started. My mom took a video of them. Their wedding went great. Then, we went into the party room.

We watched Brad and Liz's first dance as married partners. They did great. We had dinner. Then, I saw Mark and Liz dance. They were happy. Then, Brad and his mother Nancy danced. They were happy also.

Then, everyone started dancing. I danced a few times myself. I had a great time dancing. Then, we went back to the room to sleep.

On the next day, we went to Sunday brunch. It was our last day in town. We had a wonderful time. Afterwards, we went back to Miami Beach. On the next day, we went back to California.

I went back to Northern California for Alicia's 8th Grade Graduation. My mom took a video of her graduation. Marlena, Tyler, and Joey were waving in the video. Alicia got a diploma. She was going to high school in the fall. We went back to Michelle's house for her party.

On the next day, we went to the pool at the hotel, and then we went to the park with Tyler and Marlena. On the next day, I went back home.

A few days later, my mom and I went to Adventure City. It is a small theme park in Anaheim. Erika, Tyler, Nana, and Marlena were there. They rode on the kids rides. We rode on the train and pet the animals. We had a load of fun.

On July 4th, I went to Tyler's house to celebrate America's Independence Day. I brought my scooter. We went to Rancho Santa Margarita Lake to see the fireworks. We brought Dutch (Tyler's dog) with us, but the fireworks scared him very much. We humans had a wonderful time though.

On July 10, we took Tyler on the Amtrak train to Oceanside. He loved it. One strange thing happened: Tyler looked out of the window at one point and saw multiple butts outside. It was very funny, but not very cool. We arrived in Oceanside and then waited for another train to go back to Irvine. The train was packed full. We had a good experience.

On July 19, Lindsay, Danielle, Debbie, Tyler, Erika, my parents, and I got onto Kevin's boat. Kaptain Kevin drove. He was cruising around smoothly until we reached the ocean. He started driving wild, and the boat started jumping. I flew. I didn't know that I had neither a seat belt nor a vest. I hated this. Kaptain Kevin calmed back down after a while. It was an adventurous ride.

On my 34th birthday, Tyler and Brittany came to celebrate with me. Sister Linda and Justin came back to California and we went to Huntington Beach to shop and see the U.S. Open of Surfing tournament. It was very crowded. I had a great birthday weekend.

On July 29, Debbie and Nana came to see Linda and Justin. Our Scottish relatives also came to visit my Grandma Mamama. William (everyone calls him Billie) and his wife Dottie and their grandkids Kate and Jenni arrived via the metro train. Willie is my Grandma Mamama's younger brother. We went to the senior home and cafeteria with Mamama. We had a wonderful reunion.

On July 30, we went to the pool for Tyler's swimming lesson. Linda tried to teach me how to swim. I was awful at it. Still, we had a good time.

I went to Brittany's 3rd birthday party. She enjoyed her party very much. She was excited to see Tyler. Brittany's party featured a musician for kids and a ladybug cake! We sang happy birthday to her. It was a great time.

In September, we got to see my mom's childhood friend Maria Elena from their neighborhood in Santiago de Cuba. She had since moved to Puerto Rico. Her daughter Mariela had a special job to do in California, so Maria Elena came along and visited with us. We had a wonderful time.

I rode my scooter to see my grandma Mamama. I escorted her to Albertson's market. She rode her own scooter. We had a great time. One thing went wrong: Mamama and I were waiting at a red streetlight when she suddenly rode across. As the light turned green, I rode to catch up with her so that we could ride back to the senior home together.

I stayed over with Mamama for a little while before going back home. I don't think Mamama ever noticed what went wrong.

When Halloween came, I already had a costume ready. I was a Jedi from Star Wars. I went to Mamama's Halloween Party. She was dressed as a geisha with black hair and a white face (painted to look like Chinese makeup). I laughed so hard when I saw this. The party was unimpressive though. It was boring.

Afterward, my parents and I went to Tyler's house for a night of Trick or Treat with him. He was Tigger again; Erika was Pooh again; Dutch was Eeyore again. Tyler held my hand as we walked along the path of the sidewalk. (Awww. I know, right?) We had a cold and wonderful trick or treat night.

In November, we went to Aliso Beach to fly Tyler's kite. It was fun. Cute little Tyler shared control of his kite with me. (Awwwww... I know, right?!?!) I felt like I had my own little brother- except he's my nephew. I love him.

On Thanksgiving Day, we went back to Boca Raton, FL. My Grandma Vera was dying. We went to see her, and already she could not open her eyes. We slept at Mark's house. Friday, I went back to see Grandma Vera. She spoke to my mom. She said "*Arthur.*" It was my father's middle name (and the name of one of her boyfriends.)

Then I touched my grandma's hand. She said "Alberto." I don't know how she knew it was me when her eyes were closed. I love my grandma.

Mimi, Tia Maricosa, Eli, and Tessie visited me at Mark's house. I played with Eli and Tessie. Then they went back to Miami. Saturday afternoon, I went to Tia Maricosa's house to see Junior, Ahagata, and Luz. I took videos of Eli and Luz playing with their toys. We had a good time. I went back to Mark's house.

On Monday afternoon, we went out to have lunch. We had just arrived at the restaurant when Mark got a call from the senior home. Grandma Vera had passed away. We got back in the car and drove to the senior home. Grandma Vera had gone up to Heaven. She was almost 105 years old, her birthday in January just two months away. My dad was crying out. We cried with him. When we left the senior home, we went to Connie's house. We were sad. A few days later, we went back to California.

In December, I took Tyler to see Santa Claus at Fashion Island. Tyler sat on Santa's lap and smiled at the camera. We went to the giant Christmas tree and my mom took a great picture of Tyler and I by the tree with big boxes of presents. We had a great time.

We went to Craft Art. Rosa, Josefina, and Brittany were there. A half hour later, Brittney and Garrett came. Tyler and Brittany tried their hand at carving wood, and then they made a Christmas tree by hand. Brittney did Garrett's hands. We had a fun time.

On Sunday, my parents, Mamama, Debbie, Nana, Tyler and I went to the Club 25 Christmas party. We had lunch there. There was a magician that performed for the kids. Then, Santa Claus came and gave the kids Christmas presents. We had a good time.

I went to celebrate my grandma Mamama's 87th birthday at the cafeteria in her senior home. She enjoyed her birthday with us. My mom bought a cake and we sang happy birthday to Mamama.

On December 25th, everyone came to my house to celebrate Christmas. We had a Christmas meal. We went to the living room to open the Christmas presents. I gave my father the best Christmas present ever. It was a statue of a monkey laying on its back. My dad burst into laughter when he saw it. He loved his Christmas present from me. We had one of the most wonderful Christmases ever.

Chapter Fifteen:
2005

Mark, Judy and Phil came back to California. Gary, Lindsay and Mason came to visit to see them. I played with Mason. He was a good boy. Another day, we went to La Jolla with Debbie, Jack, and Marge. We had lunch at a restaurant and enjoyed each other's company. Our foreign ambassadors went home a few days later.

My parents, Tyler and I went to the park. Tyler was acting like a screaming monster on the swing. He was very funny. My dad said, "He's a maniac!" Tyler almost flipped on the swing, turning himself upside down. He asked my dad, "Can you do it?!" My dad said "No, I ain't gonna fall over!!" Later, we went to South Coast Plaza. My dad and Tyler rode the carousel. They had great fun. Afterwards, my mom took a few pictures of Tyler and I at the fountain.

My mom turned 60 years old. We went out to a restaurant with Mamama, Amnery, Jack, and Marge. We celebrated my mom's 60th birthday together. She enjoyed herself.

I went to Tyler's fourth birthday party at his new house in Trabuco Canyon. He got his own personal playground for his birthday. Tyler has cousins named Kayla and Kodi who were present, and his uncle Scott and aunt Jamie were also there. We had a great family party.

In February, my parents and I went to Maui for Rosa's son Fernando's wedding by the beach. Before the wedding, we got a condominium in Lahaina, one that was close to the beach. We met Rosa, David, Josefina, and Brittany there. I liked to play with my cousin Brittany. My parents went off to play golf. I stayed with Brittany. We went to the market together. We noticed something strange at the market: they had no Coca-Cola. They only had Pepsi. After the market, we went back to the condo. My parents got back from golf and told us that they had a great time.

Another day, I went to sit on a bench by the water and look at the ocean. I saw a whale in the middle of the ocean. It was very cool.

Then, everybody went to Maui Pineapple Plantation. We saw a few monkeys and some pineapple. We had a good time.

On the wedding day, we drove to the private beach in Waikiki. Fernando and his bride Vanessa were getting married. It was very windy. They had a harp prepared for the wedding. Brittany was the flower girl. Fernando and Vanessa were united. Then, there was champagne and wedding cake on the beach! It was a very good wedding.

The day after the wedding, we went to Mama's Fish House restaurant and had lunch. Then, we drove to see the ocean. There were people surfing in crazy winds. On the next day, we rode the ferry to get closer to the whale. I took a few pictures of it. Brittany had a great time. Then, we went to the aquarium. We loved it.

Later that night, we went to Cheeseburger in Paradise, a restaurant in Lahaina. It was Jack's favorite restaurant. We had a wonderful dinner with David, Rosa, Josefina and Brittany. Then we walked to the shops.

On our last day in Maui, I said my goodbyes to everyone. We went back to the airport, and then we flew back to California. Home Sweet Home.

In March, my parents went to Grandma Vera's funeral in Michigan. I didn't go to the funeral. It was cold in Michigan. I stayed at home with Josefina.

Then, we went to Garrett's first birthday party. He got his first birthday cake. He seemed to enjoy this. Tyler helped open his birthday present with him. I know, so cute and sweet. We had a wonderful time.

On Easter Sunday, everyone came to my house to celebrate Easter. Kevin brought his mom Sally and his grandmother. Brittany, Marlena, Tyler, and Mason went to participate in the egg hunt at my backyard. Tyler had a bunny basket for Easter eggs. He got lots of them.

Then, he transferred his Easter eggs to his wagon. This was a smart choice, and it made sense that he had made it- Tyler was a smart boy. We had a wonderful time.

On April 4, we went to Laguna Beach Hospital. We went to the waiting room and waited for Erika's baby girl to come out. I went to the cafeteria to have my lunch. I ate, and I went back to the waiting room. Monet was born! She was a beautiful baby niece. I was glad to have another niece. Tyler was happy to have a little sister. Everybody came to see Monet.

Two weeks later, we went to Alicia's 15th birthday at Erika's house. I played with Joey, Marlena, and Tyler. I took a few pictures of baby Monet. We had a great time.

My grandma Mamama's niece Betsy (and her husband Gerry) came to visit with her. We had a great dinner together and enjoyed ourselves.

I went to Marlena's 5th birthday dinner at Downtown Disney's Rainforest Café. We had a great dinner. Marlena had the greatest birthday ever.

I went to Brittany's pre-school graduation. She was not shy on the stage. She sang proudly with the choir. Then, she got her diploma. I was proud of Brittany.

My parents and I went back to Miami Beach on Memorial Day weekend. We went to the beach with my cousins. We had a good time.

On the next day, I saw a strange boat had landed on the beach from Cuba. I saw local newscasts at the beach. I thought the people had sent the new arrivals back to Cuba.

We went to Mark's jewelry store. Mark was hilarious. He gave me a few pieces of jewelry to try on. Once I was adorned, he took a picture of me. I looked like a gangster out of a Godfather movie or The Sopranos. We went to see Judy, Liz, Brad, Paul and Connie at Mark's house. We had dinner and played a dice game with real one-dollar bills. We had great fun, but I didn't win.

Beatriz visited me at Miami Beach. Later, I went to her condo. I met her daughters Daniela and Karina. Later, Martha and her family came by. Pepin and Delia also joined us. They were all so excited to see me. I met them in the 1970s. We took a few reunion pictures. We had a great time together. Karina gave me the biggest hug ever. I am going to miss them again.

I went to Tia Maricosa's house. Junior, Javi and I went to see a movie. I think we saw *Star Wars Episode III: Revenge of The Sith*. We had a great time.

We went back to California. Linda and Jessica came to California for a week. We went to Dana Point beach. Erika, Kevin, Tyler, and Baby Monet were there. We had a great time.

Later, Lindsay, Cyndee, and Garrett came to visit us. We had a sliding box that I thought might be fun to play with. It turned out that I was right. I loved Garrett's laugh when he watched a ball roll down to the floor. We had a wonderful time.

On July 4, we went to Erika's house again to celebrate. At the front of the house, they had water slides for the neighbors. Everyone was outside. I was watching my niece Monet sleep in her basket crib. I sat down on the couch. A half hour later, she woke up. I took it upon myself to look after her. She looked at me and smiled before going back to sleep. Debbie came in to watch her, so I went outside. Everyone went to the far end of the street. That evening, we went to the lake to watch the firework show.

On my 35th birthday, Gary, Mason, Marie, Adam, Lindsay, Danielle, Debbie, Erika, Kevin, Tyler, Monet, Amnery, Mario, Bertha, Carmen, Bob, Jack and Marge all came to celebrate both mine and Marge's birthday. It was wonderful.

I went to Danielle's 21st birthday dinner at Buca Di Beppo Italian restaurant. She had a great birthday.

Mamama could no longer afford to pay for her senior home. This made me sad. She moved to Woodbridge, a small apartment. Her apartment came with a mini kitchen, and she actually loved it. I liked it too. They had a pool and spa. Tyler and I went to the pool to try it out, and we had fun. Still, I'd miss being able to ride my scooter to my grandma's senior home.

I went to see Gary's boat in San Diego. We saw the craziest boat show ever. Mason and Adam both enjoyed the show. We all had a wonderful time.

I went to Lindsay's 16th birthday and Marie's daughter Jessica's 18th birthday at Gary's house. This was a good time.

In October, I babysat Monet. Tyler had school to attend. Monet and I went to the market. I liked to push Monet in the cart. I entertained her with my funny faces and a good game of peek-a-boo. She found this to be hilarious.

We celebrated Erika's 30th birthday party at her house. Another day, we went to the pumpkin patch in Laguna Wood. Tyler went on a few rides. Debbie and Monet rode the mini train.

My parents went to Club 25's Halloween party. I couldn't help but laugh at them. My mom was Martha Stewart, with a fake ankle bracelet. My dad was Donald Trump before the presidency, and his favorite quote was, "*You are fired.*" They had a great time.

I went to Erika's house to trick or treat. I was Captain Jack Sparrow. Tyler was a cowboy, namely Woody from *Toy Story*. Monet was a pink kitten. I brought my scooter with me. We went out to trick or treat. We had a great evening together.

On Thanksgiving Day, we celebrated Thanksgiving at my house. Debbie, Jay, Nana, Erika, Kevin, Tyler, Monet, Rosa, David, Brittany and Josefina came. My mom picked up Mamama and brought her to my house. Tyler and Brittany were playing and running through the grass. I took a few pictures of them. We had the most wonderful Thanksgiving ever.

I went to Lindsay's first dance performance at her high school. She danced very well. I enjoyed it.

I went to pick up Tyler and then went to Club 25's Christmas party. Debbie, Nana, Gary, Marie and Mason were there. They had the same things from last year, 2004. There was a magician and Santa Claus had presents for the children. We had a good time.

My mom, Erika, Monet, Tyler and I went to Craft Art. Rosa, Brittany and Josefina were there too. We made hand-carved Christmas ornaments from pieces of wood. We had great fun.

Christmas at my house had to be celebrated early for Alicia, Joey, and Marlena. I was eating my dinner in the kitchen. Alicia walked into our house carrying Monet. Monet saw me and got so excited that she started screaming with joy and bouncing in Alicia's arms. I smiled and finished my dinner.

Then, we opened Christmas presents. Tyler got a drum set. Monet got a rocking chair with her picture on it. Then, they went out to a movie. I had to stay in and babysit Monet. I played with her toys with her. After the movie, Monet got picked up and went home. It was a good night.

I went to pick up Tyler and Monet and we went to Brittany's Christmas Party. Debbie and Marlena were there. Santa Claus came from the North Pole for the party, but Monet was frightened by him. My mom saved her. Brittany threw a great Christmas party.

On Christmas Eve, I went to Gary's house to celebrate Christmas. We had a good dinner. We gave out presents and opened our own presents. I got $50 cash from Gary. I gave him an Elvis Presley phone. We had a wonderful Christmas.

Chapter Sixteen:
2006

In January, Billie and Dottie came back to California to visit with my grandma Mamama and the rest of our family. We went to Crystal Cathedral in Anaheim and had a wonderful time together. While they visited, I gave Billie and Dottie the chance to read the first draft of the story of my life. They told me that they enjoyed it. After a while, they went back to Scotland.

I went to Tyler's 5th Birthday Pirate Party at Pirate's Dinner Adventures in Buena Park. It looked like Medieval Times. Tyler's team won the action-packed pirate show. We all enjoyed the performance. Then, we went to Tyler's house to celebrate his victory with a cake made in his honor. He had the best birthday ever.

I went to Mason's house for his 2nd birthday party. Mason let Tyler and I join him in playing with his train tracks. We all sang "Happy Birthday" to Mason. It was a great party.

I went to see Lindsay's second dance show. She was great. This was both her second and her last one. I enjoyed the show.

We went to Disneyland with Tyler, Brittany, Rosa and Josefina. We wanted to ride in the Columbia boat. We had a great time aboard.

The young ones took a picture with Tigger before we all got on the Pirates of the Caribbean ride. I thought the drop was fun. Next, we rode The Jungle Cruise boat ride. We all enjoyed it.

Next up was Buzz Lightyear: Astro Blast. Rosa and I sat on this ride together. She scored well, but I scored even better than her. We had a "blast". Afterwards, we went to Main Street, USA to watch the parade. We had the best time.

A few days later, we went to Legoland with Erika, Marlena, Tyler, and Monet. Legoland is a Lego-themed amusement park. Marlena was acting silly, covering my eyes. My mom was able to snap a picture. Monet got excited when she saw the little Washington, DC White House. Then, Monet sat down on a Lego pig. I took a picture. Marlena got her face painted, and suddenly she looked like a fairy. Tyler got a snake painted on his arm. My dad had Monet in his care, and she cried. My mom got her, and she stopped crying. We all had a good time.

I went to Monet's first birthday party. She got a special cake. As a gift, I gave her something for the time capsule that was being assembled for her. I enjoyed Monet's birthday party.

I went to Alicia's sweet 16th birthday cruise-dinner-party in Newport Beach. Everybody came. We had a good dinner. Marlena, Tyler and my mom danced on the dancing floor. They had fun. I danced with my mom and my sister Debbie. Alicia got her birthday cake before opening any of her birthday presents. She had the greatest 16th birthday ever.

On Easter, everybody came to celebrate except Gary's family. They were on a cruise. I was playing with Monet when she saw the Easter Bunny come in. She got very scared. She ran to me and held me tight. I couldn't let Monet know that I was still a kid myself. I was afraid of Santa. Instead of blowing my cover, I saved her. I felt like Monet had my personality.

Amnery, Mario, Natalia, Brittany, Rosa, Josefina, Mike, Michelle, Alicia, Marlena and Joey came too. The Party Girl painted the kids' faces. Monet didn't get face paint because she's allergic. We took pictures of family and friends. Then, we had an Easter egg hunt in my backyard. We had the greatest Easter ever.

I went to Boomer's mini-golf theme park. We played mini-golf on the mini course. I made a hole-in-one. Joey got into a (mini) go-kart and joined the races on the track. Tyler went to the racetrack for little kids. Joey also climbed up the rock wall. He made it to the top and then fell back down. We had a great time.

Brittany had her first gymnastics show in Corona. She did well. She got a first-place trophy. I was proud of her.

On May 1st, we went to Disney's California Adventure to celebrate Marlena's 6th birthday. We had lunch at a restaurant there. Then, we went to the *A Bug's Life* attraction. I remember Monet walking near the splashing fountain. She got wet and she loved it. Then, we got on the *A Bug's Life* ride. Joey and I sat in the back, while my mom, Monet, and Erika sat up front in the bug's head. We had a great time. Then, the others rode the carousel with my dad.

We went to Soarin', my favorite ride (with a giant screen that looks like it's flying over California's coastline). Marlena had a great 6th birthday at Disney's California Adventure.

I went to Lucca's baptism. Lucca is the son of Jeanina and Hernando. We enjoyed his baptism. Then, we went to my Godmother Ana Maria's house. I enjoyed spending this time with my family. Bobbie was happy to see me. We had a great time.

I went to visit Mamama at her apartment. We made a video of my grandma telling one of her funny stories. We loved the way she told it.

On July 4th, I went to Erika's to celebrate the holiday. We watched tiny fireworks from her backyard. We had a great time.

My parents, Jack, Marge and I went to Miami Beach. We rented Teresita's condo for our stay. We had a guest waiting for us inside. It was Teresita's white dog, Baby. Teresita was out on vacation. Baby loved to sleep by my legs.

On the next day, we went to celebrate Aunt Connie's 80th birthday party. Everybody went to Mark's house and waited for the party bus that would take us to the private party place. The party bus arrived, and we got on. Mark was our host. We arrived at Delray Beach Club, Delray Beach, Florida. Suddenly, Phil's girlfriend walked up to me and slapped me on my cheek for no reason! However, nobody saw this.

We entered the party room and I got a table with Jack, Marge, and my parents. The party started and we all took pictures with Connie. Mark, Phil, Paul and I had a funny photo shoot together. We looked like the four stooges.

We ate lunch and people shared memories they had with Connie. After lunch, we sang "Happy Birthday" and ate cake. It was a great party. We took the party bus back to Mark's house. When we got to the condo, Baby peed on Jack's shoe. I laughed.

On the next day, I went to Miami to visit my cousin Mimi's family and my cousin Junior's family. Junior and Ahagata had a baby boy named J.J. He was 5 months old. He is the younger brother of Luz. We went to the movie theater to see Shrek 2 with Eli, Tessie, Luz, Mimi, and Junior. We enjoyed the movie. When it was done, I went back to the condo.

A few days later, I got a nasty cough. I went to the ER in Miami Beach. I spent 6 hours there. I did not feel good. My mom got me some medicine. She also found an air purifier machine and set it up for me. After a while, I stopped coughing and felt a little better. We went back to California.

We were planning to go to Michigan for my birthday. Before we went, we stopped by my grandma's apartment. Inside, we found my grandma on the floor- she had fallen down between the living room and the kitchen. She had forgotten to use her emergency alert necklace to call for help.

My Mom and I worked together to find someone to watch out for my grandma until we got back from Michigan.

I've forgotten until now to mention that Totica was moving to the apartment next to Mamama's. I visited my grandma and Totica often. I also forgot to mention that I had hippie hair this year. It hung down to my shoulders.

On my birthday, we went to Michigan. My sister Linda picked us up at the airport and we went to her house for the first time. Linda's house was in Lincoln Park. When we got there, Don was happy to see us. They had two good dogs. It was a strange house. They had a lot of dining rooms, one like a country booth, and many interesting rooms. Every place in the house had a tv. I met their huge and creepy fake butler. Later, Justin and Elizabeth joined us, and we celebrated my birthday with cake. Everyone sang "Happy Birthday". I was grateful. I slept on the sofa in the den. Linda kissed my cheek goodnight.

On the next day, we headed north to Michigan's Harbor Springs condos to visit Judy's brother-in-law Mike and his wife Mary Ellen. We drove for four to six hours with Judy, Marge and Jack in tow. We stopped by Michigan State University to pick up Jessica and got back on the road. We stopped at a few stores and went to Applebee's for lunch.

Then we got back on the road to Petoskey. Petoskey had steep hills and tight spaces that reminded me of Laguna Beach. Finally, we arrived at Harbor Springs Condominiums. It was a 3-story condo. I slept upstairs with my parents.

Next, we went to Linda's country house. It's been under construction for a long time. This house was a maze. Stepping inside, I saw many animal heads, couches, and televisions. There were two beds to my left. A bit up, there was a small kitchen connected to a dining room. This dining room featured Christmas trees and a long table. I made a right and found a bathroom and a bedroom, a laundry room, and yet another bathroom.

Then I went back to the dining room and kept straight into the living room. I opened and walked through the sliding doors. I made a left and found another room. I decided not to go upstairs and discover any more rooms.

We went outside and walked to a small house intended for guests. I saw lots of hummingbirds at the hummingbird feeder.

Justin and his first girlfriend Jackie took me on a ride on their golf cart to see their 10 acres of land. It looked like Frontierland. Justin drove safely because I was riding with him.

Still, there were many bumps, and we bounced through mud as we rode uphill and downhill. I saw a river, blueberries, and a few houses. Then we went back to the country house and had dinner. We had a great time with our family. Afterward, we went back to the condo.

On the next day, we went shopping in Petoskey. I was afraid that I'd fall and roll down the hill. My dad, Jack and Justin played golf. We went to Chico for my mom and Marge. I sat down on the chair with my T-Mobile Sidekick cell phone to surf the internet and watch my favorite tv shows from back home. We went and had lunch before heading back to the condo. The guys came back from golf soon after we had returned.

That evening, we went back to Linda's country house with Mary Ellen, Mike, Judy, Jack and Marge. I saw a real deer in the forest to the right of the road. At night, we went to the musical playhouse. It was a good and funny show, and when it was done, I got to meet the players. Afterwards, we went back to the condo.

On the next day, we went to Harbor Springs and went shopping. There was beautiful scenery, and there were a few boats on the lake. They have cute houses in Harbor Springs.

We went back to the condo and I had lunch. After lunch, we went to Bay Harbor to take a ride around the lake on Don and Linda's boat. We enjoyed the boat ride. We saw houses and a seaplane. The lake was huge. One of Don and Linda's dogs was afraid to ride on the boat. Jessica and Justin didn't share the fear- they jumped right in the lake. Apparently, the water was cold.

We got back to Bay Harbor and went to Boyle City, which looked almost like a New Orleans-style place. We went to a restaurant for dinner and had a great time. Then we went back to the condo. We went over to Mike and Mary Ellen's condo to visit with their family. We had a great night.

On Saturday, we got back on the boat to go to some special place with a restaurant and take a few pictures of everybody, including Jack, Marge, Judy, Mike, and Mary Ellen. I was asleep for most of this part of the trip.

Then we got back on the boat to go back to Boyle City. Later in the night, we went to Linda's country house for our last dinner there. Then, we went outside to the campfire as a family. We took a few pictures together and had a great time.

On Sunday, we were back on the road to Linda's house in Lincoln Park. We stopped at some stores in the middle of Michigan, never staying off the road too long, and finally, we arrived at Linda's house.

We went to Michelle's house to visit her family. I saw a Christmas tree in the living room. I met her son Michael and her daughter Graciella. I also met her husband Garo. Michelle made a birthday cake for me. We had a great time.

That Monday was our last day in Michigan. Lori and Chase visited in the morning. We had lunch before going to the airport. We flew back to California. Michigan was a great time.

I searched for a new nursing home for my grandma Mamama. I found one in Lake Forest. We took her by to check it out and she decided to move there. The nurses there were friendly, and she was okay.

Maria Elena came back to California. She called me "Mi Príncipe". She seemed to love makeup. We went to see my grandma. Then we went to a restaurant in Newport Beach. We had a great time. Maria Elena's daughter picked her up afterward.

Tia Maricosa came to California to help my grandma sort the things from her apartment that she wanted and sell the extra stuff. I kept her statue of Alejo and her pug pillow. From then on we started visiting my grandma daily.

On Sunday, we took my grandma out to the Catholic church festival next door to her new place. We saw some kids wearing flower leis perform a cultural song and dance routine. We had a good time. We went back to the nursing home.

By the way, Carmen was a part of the choir at this church. She made sure to visit my grandma regularly. After a while, Tia Maricosa went back to Miami.

Cousin Junior's family came back to California. We went together to visit our grandma Mamama. We had a great time with her. Then, we went to Disneyland together. Ahagata and I waited at the front castle with Luz for the fireworks to start. We had a blast. Then, we went to the swap meet (OC Marketplace). Luz went to play at the kids' house with the mini kitchen, decked out with its own refrigerator and windows. J.J. was a good baby boy in the stroller. A few days later, they went back to Miami.

In October, we went to see my sister Debbie's red hat fashion show at a hotel party room. Nana wore the red hat. We enjoyed the dinner and the magic. Then, the red hat began the show. I saw my sister Debbie come out with big hair and a red hat. She looked like the songstress legend Diana Ross. She was excited to perform, and I was proud of my beautiful sister. We took a few pictures with her afterward and went outside for a big photoshoot before going home. We had a great time.

I went to see Tyler's first karate lesson in Mission Viejo. He did well! I enjoyed watching him.

Cousin Mel-Marie came to California for a hospital conference, so we picked her up and she stayed with us. The next day, we visited our grandma Mamama. We had a great time together. The day after that, we dropped her off at the airport so that she could fly back to Alabama. I enjoyed seeing my cousin.

On Halloween, we went to Tyler's house. I was dressed as Captain Jack Sparrow from the Pirates of the Caribbean movie. Tyler was Davy Crockett. Monet was a very cute Heffalump elephant. We went out to trick-or-treat. Though it was cold, we had a good night.

On Thanksgiving Day, Debbie, Jay, Nana, Gary, Marie, Mason and Lindsay came to celebrate the best Thanksgiving dinner together. We had a great Thanksgiving.

On the next day, we took a road trip to Arroyo Grande, California. The drive took 4 hours. Arroyo Grande is in Central California. Rosa had gotten a big new house there. It was in the country near the train tracks. Brittany was too excited to see me. We stayed over at their house until the following Monday.

That Saturday, we went to Hearst's Castle. My mom and I took a special bus and she rented a wheelchair for me. Hearst's

Castle was one of the biggest museums I'd ever seen. Inside, they had what had to be the record for the biggest pool ever. We went thru the kitchen to the dining room and waited for my dad, Rosa, Josefina, Brittany and David from another bus tour.

Once they arrived, we joined up for the tour of the castle. It was very spectacular. We went to the guest house nearby. It's a small historical house. Then we went to the theater near the castle. We had a great time in this place. We got back on the road and went to see the seals on the beach. Then we went and had a late lunch at a restaurant before heading back to Rosa's house.

On Sunday, we went to the Old Mission church in San Luis Obispo. Then we went to the fish market. It was very windy out, as freezing as could be. We had a grand time. The next morning, we went to drop Brittany off at the Old Mission School in San Luis Obispo. We peeked inside of her school and prayed to have a good day. Then, we went to a restaurant for breakfast with Rosa, David, and Josefina. Then we drove four hours back to my house. I had a good time on this trip.

The following Saturday, we went to South Coast Plaza in Costa Mesa with Tyler, Monet, Erika, and Kevin. We waited in line for Tyler and Monet to take a picture with Santa. My mom carried Monet. The kids sat on Santa's lap. Monet was afraid of Santa, and she cried.

On Sunday, we went back to Club 25's Christmas Party with Tyler, Monet, Nana, Debbie and Erika accompanying us. We had brunch and saw a magician, and Santa gave all the children presents. We had a great time.

On Christmas, everybody came to my house to celebrate the best Christmas ever. Then, on December 26, we went to the airport to pick up my sister Linda, Justin and Jessica so that they could spend time with us for a week.

On my dad's 76th birthday, we all went to see Disney on Ice at the Honda Center. It was a great show. Then we went to Chuck E. Cheese to celebrate my father. We had a great laugh of a time, and we took a few pictures. I think Danielle's camera had a picture of the whole family. Well, congratulations. You made it through the longest chapter ever.

Chapter Seventeen:
2007

On New Year's Day, we went to Erika's house before driving to see the Rose Parade floats. Debbie, Michelle, Alicia, Marlena, Erika, Monet, Tyler, Linda and Jessica all came. There were too many people there! We got a few pictures of our family. We saw a Star Wars float with a live Darth Maul. Alicia and Marlena took a picture with Darth Maul, and so did I. We enjoyed all of the floats and had a great day.

On the next day, we went to the Griffith Observatory in Los Angeles with Kevin, Erika, Tyler, Jessica, Justin and Linda. I took a picture of the Hollywood Sign. We watched a film about space in IMAX. Then, we went outside to an outstanding view of L.A. I took the greatest picture: a snapshot of Tyler with that same outstanding view of L.A. behind him. We went back inside to see more science things. We saw the statue of Albert Einstein. We took a few pictures with him. He and I made Double Albert.

Then, we went to Hollywood and ate late lunch at the Hard Rock Café before walking around near the Dolby Theatre. We took a few pictures of Linda, Tyler and I on the lounge chair outside. We had a great day.

On the next day, we went to the Crystal Cathedral with Linda. We had a good time. Jessica, Justin and Linda went back to Michigan a few days later.

I went to take an allergy test. The doctor gave me a bunch of shots in my left leg. I started to feel itchy. A few days later, I got the worst chicken pox ever, all over, even in hidden places, including my balls. My balls had even swollen up some! It was extremely painful. I got an ice bag for my balls, and they stopped hurting so much. I missed Tyler's 6th birthday party while I was out of commission, but my parents were there in my place. Two weeks later, I was back to normal.

A few weeks later, I took Tyler to Disney's California Adventure for his belated birthday present. We went to Disney Animation to learn how to draw Goofy. My mom drew Goofy very well. Tyler and I did not draw what one would call a "perfect" image of Goofy. Then, we rode the Monster's Inc. ride. It was new, taking the place of the old Hollywood Stars ride. Afterward, we took a picture of us at the letter "A" in CALIFORNIA. We had a great time together.

We went to Mason's 3rd birthday party. There was a jumper. He loved bouncing around inside. We sang happy birthday and Mason opened his presents. It was a great time.

We went to the train station to pick up Brittany and Josefina so that they could spend the weekend with us. Rosa came to spend time with us as well. My parents were off to New Orleans and to take a cruise to Central America. Brittany and Rosa went back home so that Brittany could go to school. Josefina stayed over with me, and I had a great week with her.

Josefina and I rode the bus to pay a short visit to my grandma Mamama at the nursing home. We had a great time. A few days in, my parents returned from vacation. That weekend, Rosa and Brittany came back to pick up Josefina. My mom gave Brittany a gift from New Orleans. It was a mask. She liked it. After spending some time with us, they went back home.

On Easter Day, we went to Monet's house for her 2nd birthday party. There were animals in the backyard! There were sheep, baby goats, rabbits, ducks and chickens. I took a few pictures. Monet loved petting the bunnies. We sang happy birthday, and then the kids went to hunt Easter Eggs at Monet's front yard. They had a good time. Then, Monet opened her birthday presents. I enjoyed her birthday party and Easter.

Lori and Chase came to California for the first time. We celebrated Mother's Day brunch with our family. Then, we went to Balboa Island. We took a ride on the electric boat. Kaptain Kevin drove. We had a good time. Afterward, we went to Disneyland, with Kevin, Erika, Monet and Tyler tagging along. We rode the train, It's a Small World, Buzz Lightyear and Casey's Train from the movie *Dumbo*. Then, we went to Mickey's house and took a picture with him. We had a great day.

On the next day, we took Lori and Chase to see Laguna Beach. We walked to the ice cream shop for Chase. On the next day, they went back to Michigan. We haven't had a visit from them since.

We went to Lindsay's graduation dinner. I was very proud of her. Dinner was great. A few days later, Aunt Connie came to California. We went to the Santa Monica Pier and ate at a restaurant with her friend from Bakersfield. A few days later, we picked her up and went to former-President Ronald Reagan's Library. It was even bigger than Nixon's Library. We took a few pictures of the Berlin wall, statues of Ronald Reagan, and his Air Force One. I was interested in his Air Force One, so I had a look inside. It had a shower! We had a pleasant but long day. When we were spent, we went back home.

One night, my family was playing the continental card game. Connie said, "Are trio and escalera Spanish words?" My dad answered, "No! It's English!" He was serious. My Mom explained where those words came from as we all laughed.

After a good while, Connie went back to Florida.

In July, we went back to Miami Beach and rented a condo off of Collins by the beach near Publix Supermarket. We walked to the beach almost every day. Sometimes in the evening we'd walk a few blocks to eat dinner at a restaurant. One day, we went to cousin Epe's house for a family reunion. We had a great time.

Maricosa's family had been away. When they came back to the beach, we had fun with our cousins. I met cousin Mimi's baby Danny. He was a good baby. Eli and Tessie were happy to see us.

We went to Mark's house to see Connie, Paul, Liz and Brad and Penny. We had a good time. On the next day, we flew to Michigan. We stayed at Linda's house.

We drove back up north to the Harbor Springs Condo with Judy, Jack and Marge. Mary Ellen and Mike were there also.

We went back to see Linda's country house. I had a look inside. Their living room had become a sports bar with double TVs, and there was a statue of *E.T.* atop the main mantle in their living room. I liked it. On the next day, my dad, Jessica, Linda and I went to play tennis at the tennis court. I watched them play. The match was my dad and Linda versus Jessica. They were funny and fun to watch.

Judy, Marge, my mom and I went to see the tour of the houses in Harbor Springs. I thought the houses were cute. They kind of reminded me of former-President Nixon's house.

That Friday night, we went to The Young Americans Dinner Theater in Emmet County, Michigan. It was a spectacular Broadway-style dinner show. There were teenage and adult dancers and singers. We loved it, and we had a lot of fun. After the show, we went back to the condo. The next day, we went back to Linda's house in Lincoln Park.

On Sunday morning, Don wanted to show me Detroit. I let him take me hostage. He had a camera to take pictures of me all over the city. Our first stop at a Detroit police car included a real policeman. Don took a picture. Then, we went to see Jessica's work at Maybury elementary school. Don took a picture of me at her school. We went to a casino in Greektown and Don took a picture of us. Then, we went to the sports event center and he took a picture of me with Joe Louis's statue.

We went out to the Detroit Princess boat and caught a view of Toronto, Canada. He took another picture. Then we went to Justin's workplace, SmithGroup. Don took another picture. We went to the Detroit Tigers' baseball stadium and he took another picture of me. I felt like a supermodel in Detroit.

We went to Downtown Detroit and the Hard Rock restaurant. We took a few pictures outside of and inside of the restaurant. Don also took a picture of a store cashier with me. Then, we went to see the church that Elizabeth would be married at the following year: The Cathedral of Most Blessed Sacrament. He took a few pictures of me and the church.

Interestingly enough, we found our next stop by following the big sign for the gentleman's club, Club Venus. Don took a picture of me out front. Then, we went to the real strip club, Pantheion. We went inside. It was dark, dimly lit by a few neon lights. Don asked the huge bodyguard to find two strippers for a picture with a special guy. We went to the ladies bathroom to wait for the strippers. The strippers joined us, and we took a few pictures with them. It was the most embarrassing moment ever.

Finally, we went back to Linda's house. We had taken *too* many pictures. I would never forget this day.

We went to Michelle's house. I saw Michael and Graciella. We had a good time with them. On the next day, we went to downtown Detroit and ate at a restaurant with Linda's family. On the day after that, we went back to California.

In the late summer, we went to Laguna Beach with Debbie, Erika, Kevin, Tyler, Monet, Michelle, Mike, Marlena, Joey, Alicia and Danielle. I enjoyed watching them have fun in the sun. I thought it was cute when Monet played with her Grandpa Norm and I. Tyler and Marlena got in the ocean (and got out too, thank goodness!) We had a wonderful time.

We took Tyler and Monet to the pumpkin patch. We took a few pictures of Tyler, Monet and me. Then we saw the baby animals. There was a pig, a lamb, sheep and goats. We had fun.

We went to Cousin Ivette's wedding. Her husband Nick is a good man. Their wedding went perfect. We watched them dance. I had a good time.

My parents celebrated their 25th Anniversary. They went back to Carmel, and I stayed at Erika's for three days. I slept with Tyler. In the middle of the night I heard Monet crying, but I couldn't get out of the bed. Tyler was asleep on an air mattress.

One day, Erika needed to go to the bank, so I babysat Monet. She was sleeping. A half hour later, Monet wanted to pee. We went to the bathroom and she sat down on the toilet. Then, she fell in. I had failed at babysitting her! We went back to her room to play with her toys in efforts to relieve her trauma.

We saw fire at the mountains, close to the toll road 241. I had been climbing the stairs on my hands and knees, and my knees had swollen. I babysat Tyler. We watched tv and played games on my sidekick. Debbie and Jay visited us.

When they got back, my mom and dad picked me up from Erika's house on their way home. I had a great time with my family, and I'm grateful that they care for me.

On Halloween, we went to Debbie and Jay's house. Erika's family joined us. We prepared for the evening by putting on our costumes. I was a knight with a red feather hat. Tyler was a gangster with a mustache. Monet was a cute little bumblebee. Erika was a princess. Debbie was Grumpy. We went out to trick or treat in La Verne. There were too many people. We walked three blocks.

We saw Kevin's friend who was a cop. My mom and I were tired of walking, so we sat in the back seats of his cop car. We felt the hardness of the seat. It was very hard, and it hurt our butts. Afterward, we went back to Debbie's house. It was a good time.

We went to see Tyler's Thanksgiving show at his classroom. He did very well.

We went on a road trip with Erika's family to Mammoth, a six-hour drive. When we arrived at the cabin, the weather was freezing like Alaska. We went upstairs and got situated with our room, kitchen, living room and bathroom. My dad hated cold weather, and so did I. After a few hours, Michelle's family came in, followed by Debbie, Nana and Danielle. We had a full house.

On Thanksgiving Day, my family prepared turkey and other foods. I was watching Macy's Thanksgiving Parade in the bedroom. Joey and Tyler taught the family how to play the video gaming system. We had a great Thanksgiving Dinner. Afterward, we played Phase 10 and Money Train. We had a great time.

We went to the ski resort the following day. We took some great family pictures at the Mammoth statue. A lot of my family went skiing. My parents and I watched Monet. We also watched Tyler's skiing lesson.

Tyler was very good! Erika, Kevin, Mike, Michelle, Danielle, Alicia and Joey went skiing a few times. We went to the village shops and to a restaurant with Jay, Debbie, Nana, Marlena, Tyler and Monet. My mom took a picture of Monet holding my hand as we walked thru the village shops. It was too cute. We had lunch and went back to the ski resort where we waited for the others. Then we got another family picture in the snow before going back to the cabin.

We went back to the village for the Christmas show. Santa was there with real reindeer! We wanted to take a picture with Santa. As we waited for our turn, Tyler took a little nap on my lap. My mom took a picture. Then, we got our turn to take a picture with Santa. We took one of only the grandchildren first, and then we got some full family pictures with Santa.

Afterwards, we went to see the reindeer. Then we went to a restaurant for dinner. We had a great time. On the next day, we went back to the village shops. Tyler, Marlena and Monet all made art with paint. They were good painters. My dad, Nana and I sat down on the wooden bench, and my mom took a picture of us. Later in the night, we played money games with dice, Phase 10 and Money Train.

On the next day we went back home, following Kevin's truck thru heavy traffic. We had a great Mammoth Thanksgiving Vacation.

In December, we went to see The Young Americans' production "The Magic of Christmas" at the La Mirada Theatre, which the crew had turned into a winter wonderland. Jack, Marge and Judy were there also. There were 30 festive scene changes. It was one of the most spectacular shows I've ever seen.

On December 15, Mamama turned 90 years old. We celebrated her birthday with balloons shaped like "9" and "0" at her nursing home.

We went to Gary's house on Christmas eve to celebrate Christmas with his family. We had a lot of fun. I gave Gary a Nascar car collection for Christmas. On Christmas Day, we went to Erika's house with Debbie's family. We had a great Christmas time together.

Chapter Eighteen:
2008

We went to LAX to pick up Mark and Judy. Then we went to see the Christmas lights in Newport Beach and at the Trinity Broadcasting Network in Costa Mesa. My mom took a picture of my dad, Mark and I in front of the TBN building. We went inside and were greatly impressed. It was beautiful, adorned in the most impressive Christmas decorations I had ever seen. We had a look at their museum, their studio and their gift shop. It was all wonderful. On the next day, we went back to LAX. Mark and Judy went to Hawaii for a few days. They returned to California for one more day with us before heading back to Florida.

We went to see Mason's basketball game. Before the game started, Grandpa Norm taught him how to shoot the ball into the basket. Mason enjoyed this. Garrett played in another basketball game after Mason's. He was cute, and he did great. We enjoyed watching them play. On Tyler's 7th birthday, we went to see his school play before meeting at his house to celebrate. It was great.

My dad and Kevin built a playhouse for Monet in Kevin's backyard. Monet's playhouse was decked out with fantasy-style windows, a ladder leading up to her vacation bed (which sat on a second floor, mind you), a couch, a kitchen set, its own electricity, and its own doorbell. She loved it. My dad lined the outside with bricks.

One day, my dad and I went to Erika's house to finish the floor block. A few minutes in, he suddenly wasn't feeling well. His heart was beating very fast. We decided to go to the ER at Saddleback Hospital. I was afraid at the thought that my father needed to get to the hospital urgently. At one red light, my dad saw that the way was clear, so he decided not to wait for the green. My mom was waiting there for us when we arrived. We stayed at the hospital for three hours.

We got on a ferryboat to watch the whales in the southern California ocean with Tyler, Monet and Erika. We saw dolphins and whales shoot water from their heads. We had fun.

We went to Mason's 4th birthday party. He had Spider-Man decorations. There was a great magic show with a giant balloon, so giant that a man could fit inside. Actually, they did fit a man inside! We gave Mason a bike. He was happy to have it. We had a great time at Mason's birthday party.

We went to Lucca's 2nd Birthday Party at the Woodbridge Lake building. I saw my cousins Ivette, Lisette, Johnny and all of the rest of my California cousins. We had a good time.

We went to Garrett's 4th birthday party. We sang "Happy Birthday" for him. He had a wonderful birthday.

Marlena stayed with us over her Spring Break. Tyler and Marlena went to the pool at Totica's apartment. We had a special time together.

On Easter, everybody came to my house. We celebrated Nana's Birthday. Monet was playing with bubbles, trying to blow them at me. Then she'd wipe her bubble hands off on my shirt. I laughed. Garrett, Mason, Gary, Marie, Rob and Brittney came too. We had a great Easter.

We went to see Tyler's first soccer game. I watched him kick the ball to his teammate. He was pretty good at soccer. I enjoyed watching him play. We also went to Tyler's first running fundraiser at his school. He did 11 laps. I was proud of him. Around the same time, we celebrated Monet's 3rd birthday. She seemed to have a great time.

I went to Tyler's Karate tournament. He did very well. I felt proud of him. He got a cool skill under his belt.

We went to see Monet's first ballet and tap class. We enjoyed watching her. She was excited, and very cute with her tapping. She also rolled over and walked like a monkey. I took a video. We had a good time. Another weekend, we went to Dana Point Beach with Marlena, Tyler and Monet. Monet came to me to take a picture of us. I enjoyed the kids and had a good time watching them. We had a great time together.

I had a strange pain in my back around my right shoulder blade. We went to UCLA to see a doctor for my back. We didn't like this doctor. We went to San Clemente to see a different doctor, and he said that I needed to build muscle at my back and right shoulder so that I could be ready for surgery in October (a day before Elizabeth's wedding in Michigan).

We went to the Grand Opening of the Great Big Orange Balloon at the park in Irvine. It was a festival, and there were many foods. Erika's family was there. Monet flew a kite. We had a great picture taken behind the huge orange balloon ride. We did not get on the balloon ride. Still, we had a great time.

We spent July 4th at Erika's house. Tyler had set mini golf up in the backyard. My dad taught Tyler how to putt. We played mini golf together. It was a lot of fun. Later, we all watched the fireworks show at Rancho San Margarita Lake. It was beautiful.

We went back to Miami Beach. We stayed at the same Collins condo as before. We went to the beach with our cousins. Then, we walked around the Aventura mall.

One night, Mark and Judy came down to Miami Beach. We walked to Sazon's Cuban restaurant, with Tia Maricosa in our company. Yuyi, Eric and Jason were also there. We had a great dinner.

After dinner, I was walking back to the condo with Tia Maricosa when I felt my pants fall to the sidewalk. I was standing in my underwear. Tia Maricosa yelled *"Cabe!"* and we laughed. My mom fixed my pants for me and tied them up well. I was terribly embarrassed. It was the first time this had happened to me.

A few days later, we went to Mark's house and celebrated mine and Connie's birthdays. We went to a restaurant with a dance floor. We all danced together (that means me too!) and sang "Happy Birthday" for Connie and me. We had a blast of a time.

On my birthday, I went to Mimi's house to celebrate my 38th birthday. My cousins came and joined us there. Everybody sang "Happy Birthday". Mimi brought the birthday cake. I had the greatest birthday ever.

A few days later, we went back to California.

We went to Disneyland with Erika's Family. Monet got a cute Snow White outfit. We went to "Buzz Lightyear's AstroBlast", a shooting game and ride. Tyler was paired against me on the ride. Monet and my mom teamed up against my dad. We had a lot of fun.

I went back to the doctor. I had an open hole on my back shoulder. I got preemptive treatment before the surgery in October.

Before my surgery, we packed our suitcases for our trip to Elizabeth's wedding, which was in three days. On the day of my surgery, we went to Huntington Beach Hospital early in the morning. The surgery went well, and I went home in the afternoon.

Late that evening, we went to the airport to fly to Detroit, Michigan. We arrived in Michigan early in the morning. Linda picked us up from the airport. When we got to our hotel room, we found a surprise: there was a train track right next to the hotel. I heard what I thought was the loudest train horn ever. We laughed and made ourselves determined to sleep thru it.

In the early morning, we heard the *actual* loudest trains ever, at 6 am and at 8 am. Then, we went to Linda's house for breakfast. I was very tired. My mom gave me a pill and I went to sleep on the couch in the piano room, which had Halloween decorations. At 11am, My mom woke me up. We went to the reception room to set up the wedding decorations for the next day and get the tables ready.

Then, we practiced for their wedding. Afterward, we went to the Red Wings' Hockeytown restaurant for dinner. Don got some hockey pucks with Elizabeth's and Steve's names on them, and he also got everyone baseball caps celebrating University of Michigan football and embroidered with "Liz & Steve" on one side and the date of their marriage on the other.

It turned out that Robin Williams had a comic show next door at the Fox Theater. I didn't see the show. I did see many people in the lines outside. We had a good dinner with family and friends. There was a lot of traffic outside and the parking lot had become a zoo, presumably thanks to Robin Williams's show. We eventually managed to make our way to the hotel. I heard the train rumble by as I drifted to sleep.

We heard another train in the morning. Linda picked us up to ride with her. We went to Linda's house and got ready.

In the middle of the afternoon, the photographer came and took a few pictures of Elizabeth, then her direct family, and then us. We went to the church, and Steve and Elizabeth were married. It was a very special ceremony. (Andiamos in Royal Oak)

After the wedding, we went to dinner. Elizabeth looked beautiful. She mentioned how I had just had a surgery two days ago. I slow danced with the bride and with my sister Linda. Everything went great. After dinner, we helped to clean the room before heading back to the hotel.

On the next day, I woke up at 6am. I laughed as I listened to the train. I went back to sleep until 8am, when I heard another train pass by with the loudest horn yet. Then Linda picked us up and took us to her house for breakfast. Then, we went to brunch in honor of Elizabeth and Steve. We had a great time.

We went to another hotel closer to the airport. On our way, my dad talked about how happy he was to be away from the trains. We got into our room- and then I heard another train pass by, this time accompanied by an airplane. We couldn't help but laugh. My mind said, *"Seriously, another train track near the hotel, and now an airplane too?"* We said goodbye to Linda and told her we'd see her soon, and then we went to sleep until 5am. We got up and went to the diner and ate breakfast.

Then we went to the airport via the bus. We went back to California, where we'd finally be free from Michigan's trains.

My parents had a Halloween party to attend. My mom was a mistress-lady-of-sorts. My dad was a jailbird, donning an orange prison costume with fake black hair and fake shadow. He had black glasses and a scar on his face. We all enjoyed a laugh together before they set out for the party.

133

In the end of November, my mom and I went to see aunt Bobbie at her apartment. She wasn't doing well. Godmother Ana Maria, Fido and Tati were there. Aunt Bobbie's maid saw Tata's spirit in her bedroom. We were all shocked by this. On November 26, my mom gave a special prayer. We joined our hands and prayed together. Bobbie passed away at 95 years old. I was sad. I sat down in the chair and I started to cry. I felt her leave. My cousins were there in the living room.

A few days later we went to her funeral. It was sad. Bobbie had always told me *"Tu este mi corazón."* You're my heart. I will never forget her in mine.

In December, we went to see The Young Americans' Magic of Christmas. We brought Rosa, Brittany, Josefina and David with us. They added penguins this year, reminding me of the film *Happy Feet*. It was spectacular. We had a magical time.

We went to Monet's Christmas Ballet and Tap show. She was cute, yet a little confused, and that was understandable. This was her first show. All things considered, I thought she did great.

On Christmas Eve, we went to Gary's to celebrate with his family. I liked the way Garrett laughed with Uncle Mason. We had a great dinner and opened up gifts. It was a great time.

On Christmas Day, we went to Erika's house to celebrate Christmas with Debbie's family. We went to the living room to open presents. Tyler got an Xbox 360 from Debbie. They hooked it up and played the dancing video game and the air guitar video game. I loved to watch them. We had a great Christmas time.

Chapter Nineteen:
2009 (and notes in the 2000s)

I got what seemed like an infection at my back-right shoulder. There was a large red lump of inflamed muscle embedded in my skin. We went to USC's hospital to meet a new doctor. He told us that he would perform surgery in June. He planned to remove the red thing and glue my shoulder skin back in place. I was to remain awake during this surgery. I went to a treatment place in Tustin where I was given an IV for before the surgery. I wouldn't feel well at times. I went to a special wound therapy center in Newport to change the medicated bandage on my back every week.

We went to celebrate Tyler's 8th birthday at his house. He had a lot of fun. Their white dog, Sofie, loved me. I played with her tug toy and threw it. She loved to play with me.

In February, Brittany, Rosa and Josefina came to my house. Brittany painted with my mom, and she did very good. She made a bottle of red wine with a half full glass. Later on, we went shopping at Fashion Island. Brittany loved to go shopping. We had a great time.

On Spring Break, we had Marlena, Tyler and Monet. Tyler and Marlena rode my scooter up and down my street. My mom took a video. Monet and I danced like Egyptians as we waited for our turns. When we got our turn, Monet sat on my lap. We drove very slowly. Marlena took a video. We had fun.

135

We went to the park and gave the ducks and geese bread. Monet didn't know how to feed them. She didn't want to get bit by a goose, so she gave me her bread instead. I threw it at a goose as Monet laughed. We had fun. We left the park and went to Totica's apartment pool. Tyler and Marlena swam, but Monet laid out on the lounge chair to soak up a tan for a bit. She walked to the huge flowerpot, which had surprisingly few flowers. I sat down on a chair with Totica. Totica gave the kids Oreo cookies before we went home.

We went to Monet's 4th birthday "Bunnies" party. There were lots of baby bunnies. Monet loved to pet them. She went to hunt Easter eggs at her front yard and had a blast. When she was done, we sang happy birthday. She had a birthday cupcake. Then, she opened her presents. We had a great birthday and great Easter all in one day.

We went to Tyler's running event at his schoolyard. He did very well, but he took a shortcut thru the grass to the path. My mom got a video. He finished running and dumped a water bottle on himself. Monet and I sat at the lounge. She smiled at me, and this made me smile. It was a cute moment.

Tia Maricosa came to California in May. We celebrated Mother's Day with Mamama at her nursing home. We had the greatest time. A few days later, she went back to Miami.

In June, we went to see Monet's ballet and tap show at University High School Theatre in Irvine. She wore a cute outfit.

She danced on the stage. We cheered her on and enjoyed her performance. After the show, we took a few pictures.

In the middle of June, we went to USC's hospital for my awake surgery to remove the red mass from my back-right shoulder. I say "awake surgery" because there was no anesthesia. I felt a little pain from a poke at my back-right shoulder. The surgeon gave me a little gas to remove the pain.

However, I was still awake. The surgeon finished and glued my shoulder shut. The surgery went well. We went home.

We went to Miami Beach at the end of July with the same plan that we'd had every summer before: Go to the beach! It was still fun. We went to Mark's house to meet Copper, Brad and Liz's new baby boy. Liz was teaching him how to swim in Mark's pool.

There was a dog named Penny at Mark's house. She sat on my lap. My mom shot a video. Penny loved to lick my face. We had a great time with Connie, Mark, Judy, Liz, Brad and Copper.

In August, we drove to Sanibel Island with Tia Maricosa's family to celebrate Junior and Ahagata's 10th wedding anniversary. We stayed in a condo. It was ok. It was raining the next day. We were all getting ready for the big celebration. We waited for Junior and Ahagata to get there. We got the room for the event, and then, they arrived. Eli, Tessie C., Danny, Luz and J.J. were ready. I was always ready. I took some pictures. Junior and Ahagata's 10th anniversary went well.

On the next day we went to the beach. The water was perfect. My family walked in low water for a mile. I took a few pictures.

In the evening, we went to the great hamburger joint, Cheeburger Cheeburger. They had a Betty Boop cartoon board. Lindsay liked Betty Boop. My mom took a picture of Betty Boop with me. We had a great time with our cousins.

One night, I was watching the finale of "So You Think You Can Dance" at Junior's condo. My mom saw blood on my shirt. I said, "*Coño!*" My shoulder was open. The glue had not held. My mom got me a first aid patch. I saw a cloud inside the room, up near the top window. For some reason, this helped me to feel like I was ok.

A few days later, we drove back to Miami Beach. On the next day, we went back to California.

We went back to USC's hospital to see my doctor. I was rather disappointed in him: He was moving to Boston. We were tired of driving to USC every month, so we went to Laguna Wood to see a new doctor. They saw the metal rod sticking out of my shoulder. The doctor told us that they'd perform surgery in January. Every week, I went to Shari at the wound therapy center in Newport so she could change my patch. I enjoyed seeing Shari.

Near the end of August, my mom and I went to Best Buy to see a new laptop we were interested in. Just as we had arrived, my mom got a call from my dad. Jack had passed away. We went back home.

A few days later, we went to Jack's funeral. I made a slide show of pictures for him. He was the greatest friend ever. I gave his family hugs. I gave a big, extra-special hug to Marge.

In October, Mel-Marie came back to California. She had a work conference. We picked her up from the conference location. She stayed with us for a few days. We went to visit our grandma Mamama. She was happy to see her. My mom, Mel-Marie and I went to the foot massager in Irvine. But I was uncomfortable with someone holding my foot in their hand. The ladies had nicer foot massagers than mine. Mine was ok. Later, I got cramps at my feet. I took a pill to take the pain away. On the next day, Mel-Marie went back to Alabama.

On Halloween, we took a road trip to Rosa's house for a Halloween picnic in her neighborhood. Brittany was happy that we came. I felt discomfort at my shoulder. Later in the evening, many of the others went out to trick-or-treat. I stayed at Rosa's house with my dad and David. Outside was too darn cold.

After a while, the others returned. My mom took a picture of Brittany and me. We had a good Halloween... Until the early morning, when their rooster woke me at 6:30 am. It was too early. I went back to sleep. At 7:00, I heard their rooster and a train from nearby in town. I went undercover- I buried myself under the covers. I went back to sleep until 8:30 am, when everyone woke up. We went to Pismo Beach for breakfast at a restaurant. A few days later, we went back home.

139

We went to see the Young Americans' "The Magic of Christmas Spectacular" in La Mirada. Danielle and Alicia came too. We loved it.

On Christmas Eve, I went to Gary's house. We had dinner. Then, we opened presents. We had a great time. On Christmas day, we went to Erika's house. We had a great time there as well.

Sometime in the 2000s, I saw the movie "Catfish". It was an exposé of online dating about fake people misleading others with dirty tricks. I tried dating online myself. I met a few women, but they also seemed to be catfish. They were always either from Ghana, Nigeria, Belize, Sweden, China, Taiwan or Russia.

Over a Skype call, I saw that one woman I was talking to was really an African man. I quit dating online. I still hope to have a real girlfriend in the future before my mom gets too old.

I didn't have a girlfriend, but Brittany would call me over Skype. She sang "Pants on the Ground" from an American Idol singer. She loved to chat with me. She got another dog, Angel. Brittany is my godsister. I always had a very great time with her.

Linda came back to California alone to visit with us for a week. We took her to the OC marketplace (which was just a fancy way of saying swap meet). We had a good time, though I did get a sunburn on my arms and half of my face. I never forgot that experience. It was spicy.

We went to my best friend Frank's party at his mom's house. His wife's name is Rosa. She was super nice. They visited me every few years. We had a blast together.

One day when Tyler was one, he was in the kitchen with Danielle and I. Tyler was afraid of the gardener's leaf-blower. He screamed like he was auditioning for a duet with Mariah Carey. We were surprised. Danielle laughed. My poor, sweet nephew.

We went to Cirque du Soleil at Irvine Spectrum with Debbie's family. It had a Chinese theme. We loved it.

Some TVs (ones with VHF/UHF and local cable with no box) became antiques. Cassette tape, laserdisc and vhs tape were also obsolete. Good Guy, Circuit City, Mervyn's, Adventure City and the Doll/Toy Museum became pieces of history as well.

Gas prices rose higher than ever, almost $5 per gallon.

3D movies came out, and they were great for a bit, but now they just annoy me...

New technologies in the 2000s include MP3 players, iPods, touch screens, smartphones, and HDTV.

I tasted four wines at the bar with one finger. I don't like bourbon or scotch. The taste is awfully strong. I like light wine, vodka and gin. They work on me just like Nyquil though.

Also, I entered Ellen's 12 days of giveaways every year; But I didn't get any giveaways. It's okay. I hope Ellen reads this.

Chapter Twenty:
The First Half of 2010,
& My 40th birthday

In January, we took Monet and Debbie to the Santa Ana Zoo. We saw all the animals. Debbie and Monet rode on the back of an actual elephant. I took a few pictures of them. They loved it. We had a good time.

Near the end of January, I had to undergo a treatment in Tustin before my next surgery, which was scheduled in Mission Viejo in early February. The nurse that helped (or at least tried to) with the treatment tried to put a needle into my vein several times before she gave up and quit. When she quit, I quit. I left.

On Tyler's 9th birthday and my mom's 65th birthday we went to a special restaurant called Fig and Olive in Newport. Everyone had a great time.

In February, I went to Mission Viejo Hospital so they could cut the part of the bar that was sticking out of my back shoulder and clean up the wound. And then, I was asleep. The surgery went well. I woke up in the ICU wearing a tubed mask, and I was incredibly thirsty. American Idol played on the tv. My parents slept in my room with me.

The next morning, I could no longer breathe with the tube over my face. I pulled, and pulled harder, and the tube popped off.

I could breathe again, but my voice had become like Darth Vader's. I waited to go to my room in the hospital.

Soon, I had visits from Bertha, Amnery, Mario, Christina, Totica's family, Godmother Ana Maria, Diana and Jeanina. They gave me balloons and flowers. Shari visited me. My parents stayed and slept there until Friday, when we went home sweet home. I had stitches that needed to be taken out next month.

In March, we visited Brittney in the hospital and met a new baby girl. She was named Kylee. She was too cute. Garrett had a baby sister now. I smiled at them. Then, we went home.

At the end of March, Javi and Lauren came to visit us. I gave Javi my "Han Solo Trilogy" books and "Empire Strikes Back" poster. Javi gave me a figure of Chewbacca. They were a super nice couple.

In April, we went to celebrate Monet's 5th birthday at her family's house. She was happy to see me. We went to Baskin Robbins' Ice Cream. She loved it. She had a great birthday.

In May, we went to Brittany's first communion at Old Mission Church. She did well. Then, we went to her family's house for a party in the backyard with a DJ and a Mexican mariachi band. I hate mariachi music. I don't know why.

Then, Brittany showed off her skills and danced like Michael Jackson. Her favorite song by Michael Jackson was Bad. A few days later, we went back home.

In June, I got a new iPhone 4, my first iPhone ever for my 40th birthday. I got a Samsung laptop from Best Buy too. My mom and I went to see the venue for my birthday party in Newport Beach. We liked it. Mamama paid for my birthday party. A few days later, we went to see a potential chef for my party. We invited him to cook for our event and he agreed. A manager at the venue told us that no physical band would be allowed. They would only allow a DJ. We were a bit disappointed by this. However, it was okay.

On the day of my 40th birthday party, Rosa, David, Brittany and Josefina arrived at my house. We all got ready to go to my party together. We arrived a bit early. Bertha was the first one there. We all went inside and placed decorations and pictures.

An hour later, everyone began to show up for my party. Everybody smiled for me, and they were excited to be there. My school friends Frank and Rosa came, and Tyler took a few pictures of us. My teacher Mrs. Charbonneau came. She was excited to see me.

We sat to eat dinner. Then, I showed a slideshow of my old pictures. Everybody laughed at the last picture of me in a speedo. Then my childhood friend Adam Crow came and stood by me. Brittany performed a dance routine to Michael Jackson's song "Bad". Adam got my iPhone 4 and recorded her performance for me. She did excellently and continued to dance to even more Michael Jackson after the first song was over. I enjoyed the dance.

Then, my brother Gary gave a great speech about me. I was proud of him. Then the DJ began. I danced with my mom. Then everybody wanted to dance with me. I agreed.

Everybody sang "Happy Birthday". I was happy. I had the greatest birthday ever. But my birthday wasn't over in Miami yet.

In July, we went back to Miami Beach. We stayed at the Collins condo. We went to Luz's first Communion. It went super great.

Then, we went to the hotel club room to celebrate her first communion with a party. We had a great time.

A few days later, Mel-Marie and Hena Te joined us from Alabama. We picked Linda and Jessica up at the airport. Then, we went back to the condo. They brought t-shirts for my birthday party the next day. This was an exciting evening.

On Saturday afternoon, we went to the club room to decorate and set up the food. Then we went back to get ready for my party, which would go on from 5pm to 8pm. Everyone came. They were excited to see me and to see our cousins. We sang happy birthday with no cake. We had a great time.

 Except the condo valet came and said, "I have an urgent problem. The parking lots are full." Someone from my party had left their car with him and he had been unable to park it. Everyone left my party at 8:30 pm. I was disappointed. We went back to the condo room with much of our family. I opened my birthday presents and was pleased. I had a good night.

Suddenly in the middle of the night, I was not feeling well. I could not breathe. I had an asthma attack. My mom helped me. We went to the kitchen. She got a pot and filled it with water. She turned on the stove and set the water over the fire. We used the steam from the hot water to open up my nose, and to help relax my lungs and calm my asthma down. I thought maybe my surgeon had poked my right lung during my surgery in early February. He did say that he had noticed air inside my right lung. Then, we went back to sleep. I felt a little better.

On my actual birthday, a tropical storm with heavy wind and heavy rain hung over us for one hour. I heard the condo's boss request over the loudspeaker that we bring all patio furniture inside and lock the sliding doors.

It was almost like a hurricane. One hour later though, things had gone back to normal. I ate my breakfast pancake with a candle. My family sang "Happy Birthday" to me again. I had a good birthday breakfast.

Later, we went on the Duck Bus Tour to see Miami Beach. The Duckbus went in the lake to show off a few celebrities houses, like Shaq, Celine Dion, Gloria Estefan and Dr. Phil. We enjoyed it. Then the Duckbus went back up onto the road.

Then, they sang "Happy Birthday". It was the last birthday song for my 40th. We went back to the condo. I had a great 40th birthday parties and birthday-Duckbus-Tour with Linda and Jessica.

A few days later, everyone went back home. I had the greatest birthday vacation ever.

Well, this is the end of my story, for now. I may work on my next book, my last book very-very-very soon. Until then, I hope that You've enjoyed the second volume. I want to give very special thanks to Tyler Koorndyk for the painting on the front cover and the picture of me, Trenton (Benard) McCullouch for editing this, Erika Koorndyk for the picture of my dad Norm Baston, and my mom Tessie Baston for everything.

Yours truly,
Alberto Baston

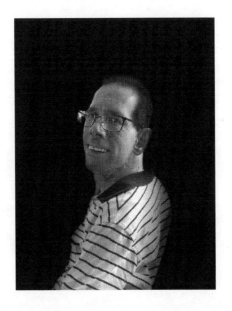

Alberto Baston lives in Irvine, California with his mother, Tessie. Alberto has spent an impressive amount of energy throughout his life documenting his experiences- as well as his family's- and making efforts to entertain and inspire the youth and to put smiles on the faces of those close to him. Alberto is an effective communicator who works every day to further overcome the challenges of being born non-verbal, and he gives a podcast on Spotify and Anchor titled *Alberto's Discourse.* He is also awesome. Follow Alberto on Instagram: @abaston. Thank You for reading!!

Made in the USA
Monee, IL
16 February 2020